THE

EVERYTHING
PREGNANCY
ORGANIZER

3RD EDITION

Welcome to the EVERYTHING® Series!

These handy, accessible books give you all you
need to tackle a difficult project, gain a new hobby,
or even brush up on something you learned back in
school but have since forgotten.

When you're done reading, you can finally
say you know **EVERYTHING®**!

PUBLISHER Karen Cooper

DIRECTOR OF ACQUISITIONS AND INNOVATION Paula Munier

MANAGING EDITOR, EVERYTHING® SERIES Lisa Laing

COPY CHIEF Casey Ebert

ASSISTANT PRODUCTION EDITOR Jacob Erickson

ACQUISITIONS EDITOR Brett Palana-Shanahan

DEVELOPMENT EDITOR Brett Palana-Shanahan

EDITORIAL ASSISTANT Ross Weisman

EVERYTHING® SERIES COVER DESIGNER Erin Alexander

LAYOUT DESIGNERS Colleen Cunningham, Elisabeth Lariviere,
Ashley Vierra, Denise Wallace

Visit the entire Everything® series at *www.everything.com*

THE
EVERYTHING®
PREGNANCY ORGANIZER

3RD EDITION

A complete, month-by-month guide
for the mom-to-be!

Paula Ford-Martin

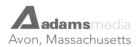

Adamsmedia
Avon, Massachusetts

Published by Adams Media, a division of F+W Media, Inc.
57 Littlefield Street
Avon, MA 02322
www.adamsmedia.com

ISBN 10: 1-4405-2676-1
ISBN 13: 978-1-4405-2676-3
eISBN 10: 1-4405-2821-7
eISBN 13: 978-1-4405-2821-7

Printed in China.

10   9   8   7   6   5   4   3   2

This book is intended as general information only, and should not be used to diagnose or treat any health condition. In light of the complex, individual, and specific nature of health problems, this book is not intended to replace professional medical advice. The ideas, procedures, and suggestions in this book are intended to supplement, not replace, the advice of a trained medical professional. Consult your physician before adopting any of the suggestions in this book, as well as about any condition that may require diagnosis or medical attention. The author and publisher disclaim any liability arising directly or indirectly from the use of this book.

This publication is designed to provide accurate and authoritative information with regard to the subject matter covered. It is sold with the understanding that the publisher is not engaged in rendering legal, accounting, or other professional advice. If legal advice or other expert assistance is required, the services of a competent professional person should be sought.
—From a *Declaration of Principles* jointly adopted by a Committee of the American Bar Association and a Committee of Publishers and Associations

Many of the designations used by manufacturers and sellers to distinguish their product are claimed as trademarks. Where those designations appear in this book and Adams Media was aware of a trademark claim, the designations have been printed with initial capital letters.

Interior illustrations by Michelle Dorenkamp

This book is available at quantity discounts for bulk purchases.
For information, please call 1-800-289-0963.

Contents

Introduction

Congratulations! You're pregnant! Once the shock begins to wear off, you're probably going to have a lot of questions about the whole process—not to mention a lot to do! But don't worry, this book is designed to help you make the next nine months as stress free as possible. It includes all the information you need to enjoy a healthy, happy pregnancy—from food and nutrition tips to what to expect at your doctor's visits.

Use the worksheets, planning calendars, charts, and checklists in these pages to keep all your essential information in one place. And take the book along with you to the many appointments you will have over the next few months.

Have fun with the calendar, and use it for every aspect of your pregnancy. It can serve as an easy reminder to know exactly what week you are in as well as a way to keep track of doctor's appointments, scheduled tests, and when to expect the results. You can also jot down your thoughts and feelings on particular days that are important to you: the day you first felt the baby kick; the day you stopped feeling queasy;

the day your regular clothes stopped fitting; your first shopping trip to the maternity store; the day you somehow "knew" just what the sex of the baby would be.

We've also included journal pages where you can record your experiences throughout each month of your pregnancy. It's a great keepsake to share with your new child one day.

PART 1

Getting Ready

After you've confirmed the good news that you're pregnant, you can begin to prepare for your pregnancy and beyond. You'll need to research healthcare provider options (from traditional to alternative practitioners), choose a healthcare provider, and begin taking prenatal vitamins to provide your baby with a healthy start.

Choosing a Healthcare Provider

Even if you have a picture-perfect pregnancy, you will be seeing a lot of your healthcare provider over the next nine months. The American College of Obstetricians and Gynecologists (ACOG) recommends that women see their providers:

- Every four weeks through the first twenty-eight weeks of pregnancy (about seven months)
- Once every two to three weeks between twenty-nine and thirty-six weeks
- Every week after thirty-six weeks

If you have any conditions that put you in a high-risk category, such as diabetes or a history of preterm labor, your provider may want to see you more frequently to monitor your progress.

Who should guide you on this odyssey? If you currently see a gynecologist or family practice doctor who also has an obstetric practice, he or she may be a good choice. If you don't have that choice, or would like to explore your options, consider the following healthcare professionals.

- **Ob-gyn:** An obstetrician and gynecologist is a medical doctor (MD) who has received specialized training in women's health and reproductive medicine.

- **Perinatologist:** If you have a chronic health condition, you may see a perinatologist—an ob-gyn who specializes in overseeing high-risk pregnancies.
- **Midwife:** There are certified nurse-midwives licensed to practice in all fifty states. They provide patient-focused care throughout pregnancy, labor, and delivery.
- **Nurse practitioner:** A nurse practitioner (NP) is a registered nurse (RN) with advanced medical education and training (at minimum, a master's degree).
- **Combined practice:** Some obstetric practices blend midwives, NPs, and MDs, with the choice (or sometimes the requirement) of seeing one or more throughout your pregnancy.

A doula is a pregnancy and birth support person who cannot replace any of the above professionals, but who can provide emotional assistance to both the mom-to-be and her family. Doulas can assist you at any point in pregnancy, from preconception to postpartum. Because doulas tend to work with a variety of physicians and midwives in many different settings, they may also be helpful in providing information on places and providers as you plan your birth experience.

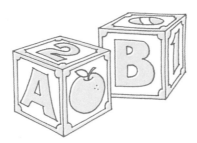

Whether it's your first or your fifth, this pregnancy is a one-time-only performance. You deserve the best support in seeing it through. Talk to the experts and get referrals. Ask for referrals from the following:

- Friends
- Family members
- State or county medical board
- Patient services department of nearby hospitals and/or birthing centers
- Labor and delivery programs of nearby hospitals and/or birthing centers
- Medical centers
- American Congress of Obstetricians and Gynecologists *www.acog.org*
- The American College of Nurse-Midwives *www.midwife.org*

On the following worksheets, record information about referrals that you gleaned from your contacts and/or local medical facilities and organizations.

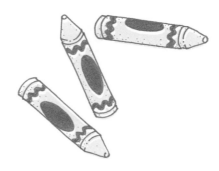

Healthcare professional's name

Position

Telephone number

Address

Referred by

Covered by your health insurance?

Healthcare professional's name

Position

Telephone number

Address

Referred by

Covered by your health insurance?

Healthcare professional's name

Position

Telephone number

Address

Referred by

Covered by your health insurance?

Healthcare professional's name

Position

Telephone number

Address

Referred by

Covered by your health insurance?

Healthcare professional's name

Position

Telephone number

Address

Referred by

Covered by your health insurance?

Healthcare professional's name

Position

Telephone number

Address

Referred by

Covered by your health insurance?

Healthcare professional's name

Position

Telephone number

Address

Referred by

Covered by your health insurance?

Healthcare professional's name

Position

Telephone number

Address

Referred by

Covered by your health insurance?

Healthcare professional's name

Position

Telephone number

Address

Referred by

Covered by your health insurance?

Once you've narrowed down your list of potential providers, it's time to find out more about them. Some providers have staff to answer your questions over the phone, whereas for others you might need to schedule a face-to-face appointment.

You can photocopy the interview questions provided here and record answers for each healthcare professional. Be sure to talk with your partner about your biggest questions, concerns, and expectations before you go.

What are the costs and payment options? If your health plan doesn't provide full coverage, find out how much the remaining fees will run and if installment plans are available.

....

....

....

....

....

....

....

....

....

....

....

Who will deliver my baby? Will the doctor or midwife you select deliver your child, or will it be another provider in the practice, depending on when the baby arrives? If your provider works alone, find out who covers patients during vacations and emergencies.

....

....

....

....

....

....

....

Who will I see during office visits? Group practices typically share delivery responsibilities. You may want to ask about rotating your pre-natal appointments among all the providers in the group so you'll see a familiar face in the delivery room when the big day arrives.

....

....

....

....

....

....

What is your philosophy on routine IVs, episiotomies, labor induction, pain relief, and other interventions in the birth process? If you have certain expectations regarding medical interventions during labor and delivery, you should lay them out now.

....

....

....

....

....

....

....

What hospital or birthing center will I go to? Find out where the provider has hospital privileges and ask for more information on that facility's programs and policies. Ask if a neonatal unit is available if problems arise after the baby's birth. Many hospitals offer tours of their labor and delivery rooms for expectant parents.

....

....

....

....

....

....

What is your policy on birth plans? Will the provider work with you to create and, more important, follow a birth plan? Will the plan be signed and become part of your permanent chart in case he or she is off duty during the birth?

....

....

....

....

....

....

....

How are phone calls handled if I have a health concern or question? Most obstetric practices have some sort of triage (or prioritizing) system in place for patient phone calls. Find out how quickly calls are returned and if your provider will be available to speak to if necessary. And since babies don't keep bankers' hours, find out what system they have in place for handling night and weekend patient calls.

....

....

....

....

....

Early Pregnancy Nutrition

From the start, your developing child requires an extra boost of a variety of vitamins and minerals. Folic acid, found in green leafy vegetables and enriched grains and cereals, is particularly important in the early months of pregnancy. During pregnancy, this vitamin helps to properly develop the neural tube, which becomes the baby's spine. When taken in daily optimal amounts during the first trimester, folic acid can help prevent birth defects of the brain and spinal cord, called neural tube defects (NTDs). This is why prenatal supplements are usually prescribed as soon as you find out you're pregnant. Here are some other essential nutrients you'll need:

Recommended Daily Intake of Nutrients in Pregnancy* (for women aged 19–50)

Calcium. . . . . 1,000 mg
Copper. . . . . 1,000 mcg
Folic acid/Folate . . . . 600 mcg
Iodine . . . . 220 mcg
Iron . . . . 27 mg
Magnesium . . . . 350–360 mg
Niacin . . . . 18 mg
Riboflavin . . . . 1.4 mg
Selenium . . . . 60 mcg
Thiamin. . . . . 1.4 mg
Vitamin A . . . . 770 mcg
Vitamin B_6. . . . . 1.9 mg
Vitamin B_{12} . . . . 2.6 mcg
Vitamin D . . . . 15 mcg
Vitamin C . . . . 85 mg
Vitamin E . . . . 15 mg

Vitamin K . . . . 90 mcg

Zinc . . . . 11 mg

*Recommended daily intake from food and supplement sources combined.

Source: Food and Nutrition Board, Institute of Medicine, National Academy of Sciences; *Dietary Reference Intake Tables*.

Changing Habits and Food Journals

Perhaps you're concerned that your nutritional intake is not up to par. Don't worry—there is time to make changes. The key is to make only a few changes at a time. Trying to change your entire diet at one time can be frustrating and discouraging. Start with simple goals—such as eating at least three meals a day, eating two servings of fruit per day, drinking eight glasses of water each day, or walking thirty minutes three times per week—and work your way up from there. Once you have mastered one set of habits, move on to the next. Be sure your goals are realistic, specific, and attainable. "Eat more fruit" is a noble goal, but it might help to make one that's more specific, like "Eat two servings of fruit each day."

To aid in your endeavors, find a way to monitor yourself, such as a food journal. Self-monitoring has been shown to help change a behavior in the desired direction. Keep in mind that it takes at least twenty-one days to actually change a habit—be patient. Use your food journal to write down everything you eat and drink throughout the day; this can help you stay committed to your goals of eating a healthier diet. Write each item down as soon as you have eaten it. That way you won't conveniently forget to take note of certain foods at the end of the day. Keep track of your exercise habits and how much water you drink, too. Copy the following food log and use it to track your progress each day.

Go to the United States Department of Agriculture (USDA) Daily Food Plans for Pregnancy & Breastfeeding at *www.MyPyramid .gov/mypyramidmoms/* for more information on healthy eating habits.

FOOD LOG

Food	Portion	Time Eaten	Activity Following Consumption
french fries	1 cup	3:15 P.M.	went for a walk

The Scoop on Prenatal Vitamins

Prenatal supplements (PNVs) are specialized vitamin and mineral supplements that women can take even before pregnancy to get all of the essential nutrients they need during pregnancy. Studies have shown that the use of prenatal supplements before and throughout pregnancy can benefit a healthy baby.

Prenatal vitamins come in many formulations. Most PNVs are distributed as samples to physician's offices, and it is a good idea to try multiple samples because some have stool softeners and other binders, which you may or may not tolerate. Finding one that you can tolerate will make it easier to take and therefore easier to remember to take daily.

The components all PNV supplements should have in common are folic acid, iron, and calcium. Most PNVs have only 100–250 mg of calcium—women need 1,000 mg daily, so you should also take a separate calcium supplement. Except for calcium, you should never take any additional supplements with your prenatal supplement unless they are prescribed by your doctor. Since some over-the-counter supplements contain too-high levels of vitamins and minerals, it may be smarter to use a supplement such as a PNV that has been specifically formulated for pregnant women and/or women trying to conceive.

Common Tests

Over the course of your pregnancy, you'll be visiting your healthcare provider quite a bit. Your provider will administer a number of tests to make sure that you and your baby remain healthy throughout your pregnancy, and that neither you nor your baby are at risk for complications.

Following are some of the most common tests you will undergo and what they test for.

Urine culture
Tests for presence of ketones and levels of protein, bacteria, and glucose

Rh factor (Rh positive or negative)
If you are Rh negative, you are at risk for Rh incompatibility with the blood type of your baby

Hemoglobin/hematocrit
Tests for anemia

Rubella
Tests for past infection with German measles if you have not previously received the rubella vaccination

Glucose challenge test
Tests for gestational diabetes mellitus

Oral glucose tolerance test
Provides definitive diagnosis of GDM

Hepatitis B
Tests for the presence of Hepatitis B in the blood

Pap smear
Detects cervical cancer, precancerous cells, vaginal infections, STDs, and inflammation of the cervix

Chorionic villus sampling (CVS)
Tests for Down syndrome and more than 200 other disorders

Alpha-fetoprotein (AFP) blood tests (or variations called the triple or quad AFP screens)
Screens for chromosomal irregularities like trisomy 18 and Down syndrome, and for neural tube defects

Cystic fibrosis screening
Screens to see if you are a carrier

Amniocentesis
Diagnoses chromosomal abnormalities, genetic disorders, and birth defects

Ultrasounds
May be used to diagnose placental abnormalities, an ectopic pregnancy, or certain birth defects

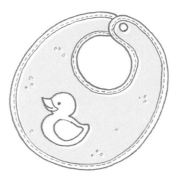

PERSONAL MEDICAL HISTORY WORKSHEET

Fill out your personal medical history here so you can easily answer the questions your doctor will ask you at your first visit.

Chronic illnesses:

....

....

....

....

....

Current medications:

....

....

....

....

Current vitamins, dietary supplements, and herbal supplements:

....

....

....

....

....

Fill out your personal medical history here so you can easily answer the questions your doctor asks you at your first visit.

Allergies to medications:

....

....

....

....

Past surgeries:

....

....

....

Tobacco use (include frequency of use):

....

Average number of alcoholic beverages consumed per week:

....

Current level of physical activity:

....

....

....

Fill out your personal medical history here so you can easily answer the questions your doctor asks you at your first visit.

Have you had:	Yes	No
Seizure disorder	○	○
Epilepsy	○	○
Insomnia	○	○
Frequent anxiety	○	○
Frequent depression	○	○
Recurrent headache	○	○
Asthma	○	○
Pain/pressure in chest	○	○
Chronic cough	○	○
Palpitations (heart)	○	○
Valvular, congenital, or other heart disease	○	○
High or low blood pressure	○	○
Rheumatic fever or heart murmur	○	○
Back problems	○	○
Tumor, cancer, cyst	○	○
Jaundice (liver disease)	○	○
Stomach or intestinal trouble	○	○
Mononucleosis	○	○
Gallbladder trouble or gallstones	○	○
Recurrent diarrhea	○	○
Hernia	○	○
Recent weight gain/loss	○	○
Dizziness, fainting	○	○
Weakness, paralysis	○	○
Blood clots	○	○
Thyroid disorders	○	○

Fill out your personal medical history here so you can easily answer the questions your doctor asks you at your first visit.

Have you had:	Yes	No
Urinary tract infections or kidney disease	○	○
Bowel disease	○	○
Significant hemorrhoids	○	○
Blood transfusion	○	○
Albumin (protein in urine)	○	○
Blood in urine	○	○
Sugar in urine	○	○
Diabetes	○	○
Peptic ulcer	○	○
Collagen disease	○	○
Pneumonia	○	○
Irregular periods	○	○
Severe cramps	○	○
Excessive menstrual flow	○	○

Sexually Transmitted Diseases   Treatment
(past and present, if any)

....

....

Fertility issues (if any)   Treatment

....

....

Fill out your personal medical history here so you can easily answer the questions your doctor asks you at your first visit.

Number of previous pregnancies: _____

In previous pregnancy, have you experienced:	Yes	No
Birth weights less than 2,500 grams	O	O
Birth weights greater than 4,000 grams	O	O
Preterm labor	O	O
Preterm rupture of membranes before onset of labor	O	O
Complications with labor or delivery	O	O
Pregnancy-induced hypertension	O	O
Preeclampsia	O	O
Eclampsia	O	O
Postpartum hemorrhage	O	O
Third-trimester bleeding	O	O
Anemia	O	O
Miscarriage	O	O
Stillbirth	O	O
Abortion	O	O
Neonatal death	O	O

Previous miscarriage or abortion   **Date of miscarriage or abortion**

....

....

Other complications during previous pregnancies   **Treatments**

....

....

FAMILY MEDICAL HISTORY WORKSHEET

Fill out your family medical history here so you can easily answer the questions your doctor asks you at your first visit.

Medical Condition	Yes	No	Do Not Know	Relationship
Diabetes	○	○	○	_____
Hypertension	○	○	○	_____
Psychiatric disorders	○	○	○	_____
Alcoholism	○	○	○	_____
Neural tube defects	○	○	○	_____
Multiple births	○	○	○	_____
Macrosomia	○	○	○	_____
Congenital defects	○	○	○	_____
Hearing problems	○	○	○	_____
Cleft palate or lip	○	○	○	_____
Sickle cell anemia	○	○	○	_____
Hemophilia	○	○	○	_____
Down syndrome	○	○	○	_____
Cystic fibrosis	○	○	○	_____
Huntington's chorea	○	○	○	_____
Cerebral palsy	○	○	○	_____
Muscular dystrophy	○	○	○	_____
Nerve-muscle disorder	○	○	○	_____
Thyroid disorder	○	○	○	_____
Other hormonal disorder	○	○	○	_____
Dwarfism	○	○	○	_____
Hepatitis B, C, or carrier	○	○	○	_____
Blindness, visual problems	○	○	○	_____
Hand or feet abnormalities	○	○	○	_____
Autism	○	○	○	_____
Miscarriage	○	○	○	_____

Fill out your family medical history here so you can easily answer the questions your doctor asks you at your first visit.

Medical Condition	No	Yes	Do Not Know	Relationship
Lou Gehrig's Disease	○	○	○	_____
Cancer	○	○	○	_____
Endometriosis	○	○	○	_____
Sudden infant death syndrome	○	○	○	_____

Other

....

....

....

....

....

....

....

....

....

....

....

PART 2

Month One

During the first trimester of pregnancy, which lasts approximately fourteen weeks from the first day of your last menstrual period, your body is hard at work forming one of the most intricate and complex works of nature. By the end of your first official month of pregnancy (six weeks after your last menstrual period, but four weeks since conception), your developing child will have grown an astonishing 10,000 times in size.

Month One Checklist

✓ Evaluate your doctor, midwife, or group practice and decide if it's right for you and your pregnancy.
✓ Discuss any possible on-the-job hazards with your doctor or midwife.
✓ Evaluate your diet and begin taking prenatal vitamins if recommended by your doctor or midwife.
✓ Get up to speed on your health insurance coverage for prenatal visits, delivery, and the care of your child.
✓ If you smoke or drink, quit now.
✓ Prepare a budget to save for when your baby arrives.

Your Baby This Month

Making its longest journey until the big move nine months from now, your developing baby (called a zygote, or fertilized ovum) travels from the fallopian tube and into the uterus (or womb). By day four, the zygote has formed a small solid cluster of cells known as a morula.

By day five or six, the morula grows to a blastocyst. Within days, the blastocyst nestles into the nutrient-rich lining of your uterus (the endometrium) as implantation begins. About fifteen days after conception, the blastocyst becomes an embryo. Next to the embryo floats the yolk sac, a cluster of blood vessels that provide blood for the embryo at this early stage until the placenta takes over.

As month one draws to a close, your baby's heart is beating, lung buds have appeared, and construction of the gastrointestinal system and liver are underway. The neural tube, the basis of the baby's central nervous system, has developed and the forebrain, midbrain, and hindbrain are defined. He (or she) is starting to look more like a person, too. Arm and leg buds—complete with the beginnings of both feet and hands—are visible. It's an amazing list of accomplishments considering your baby is about the size of a raisin (less than ¼" long).

Your Body's Changes

At this point in your pregnancy, you might not notice any significant changes in shape and size. You may feel some of the following changes, though. Note which you are experiencing so you can look back on the progress of your pregnancy and discuss any concerns you have with your healthcare provider.

— You feel slightly bloated, and your waistband begins to feel a bit snug.
— Your breasts are starting to increase in size.
— The areolas around your nipples enlarge and darken.
— Your breasts are more tender.
— Vaginal secretions increase, similar to those you get premenstrually.
— You may feel tired and run down. (Grab a nap during the day or make an early bedtime a priority.)

— You may feel faint or dizzy. (Sit or lay down on your side as soon as possible. Try not to lay flat on your back as this can make the dizziness worse.)

Morning Sickness

About three-quarters of pregnant women have morning sickness during their first trimester. Called nausea and vomiting of pregnancy (NVP) by the medical profession, morning sickness is arguably the most debilitating and prevalent of pregnancy symptoms. The following treatments have been associated with some success in lessening morning sickness.

Eat ginger. Ginger snaps and other foods and teas that contain ginger (*Zingiber officinale*) may be helpful in settling your stomach.

Try acupressure. Sometimes used to ward off motion sickness and seasickness, acupressure wristbands called Sea-Bands place pressure on what is called the P6, or Nei-Kuan, acupressure point. Available at most drugstores, they are an inexpensive and noninvasive way to treat morning sickness.

Consider B vitamins. Vitamin B_1 (otherwise known as thiamin) and vitamin B_6 have reduced morning sickness symptoms in several clinical trials. Talk with your doctor or midwife before taking any supplements.

Eat smaller, more frequent meals. An empty stomach produces acid that can make you feel worse. Low blood sugar causes nausea.

Choose proteins and complex carbohydrates. Protein-rich foods—such as yogurt and beans—and complex carbs—such as whole-grain breads—are good for the two of you, and may calm your stomach.

Eat what you like. Most pregnant women have at least one food aversion. If broccoli turns your stomach, don't force it. The better foods look and taste the more likely they are to stay down.

Drink plenty of fluids. Don't get dehydrated. If you're vomiting, you need to replace those lost fluids. Some women report better tolerance of beverages if they are taken between meals rather than with them.

Avoid strong smells and tastes. The heightened sense of smell many women experience in pregnancy can set your stomach off. Try avoiding foods with a strong odor, like fish. The same goes for spicy foods; bland is often best when you're dealing with nausea.

Brush regularly. Keeping your mouth fresh can cut down on the excess saliva that plagues some pregnant women and contributes to nausea. Breath mints may be helpful, too.

Talk to your provider about switching prenatal vitamins. Iron is notoriously tough on the stomach, so your provider might recommend a supplement with a lower or extended release amount.

Morning Sickness Survival Kit

If your stomach won't behave but you have to commute to work or elsewhere, put together a morning sickness survival kit for the car. Include the following items:

- Wet wipes
- Gum or breath mints

- Tissues
- Large freezer-grade zip-top bags
- Small bottle of water
- Graham or soda crackers
- Travel-sized toothbrush and toothpaste
- Just-in-case change of clothes

On Your Mind

Pregnancy is a time of great anticipation as you head out into uncharted waters. Worries about the baby's health and the possibility of miscarriage are common fears early in pregnancy. Although it may be easier said than done, letting go of your anxieties, at least for a little while, is the best thing for you and your baby right now.

Here are some ways to deal with anxiety about miscarriage and stress about the pregnancy:

- Designate a certain area of your home a worry-free zone, and use stress-busting strategies like soft music, aromatherapy candles, and favorite photos to create a soothing atmosphere.
- Try a prenatal massage from a licensed practitioner.
- Talk to other moms-to-be in an online pregnancy support group.
- Practice meditation and deep-breathing exercises.

Eating for Two

Once you become pregnant, you may hear comments like, "Go ahead and eat; you are eating for two now." It is true that you need nutrients through the foods you choose for both you and the healthy development of your baby. Eating plenty of nutritionally dense foods—as opposed to junk that contains calories but very little nutrition—is the way to supply your baby with all the nutrition he needs. On the other hand, you don't need to eat enough calories for two. In fact, eating too much can cause unnecessary weight gain. At the same time, eating too little may keep your baby from receiving all of the nutrition he needs. The key is to keep a healthy balance.

Calorie needs increase slightly during pregnancy to help support a woman's maternal body changes and the baby's proper growth and development. It is true that your body requires more calories during pregnancy, but "more" here means only a moderate amount. After the first trimester, you need about 300 calories per day above your maintenance level. That adds up to about 85,000 calories over the nine months that you are pregnant. Calorie needs will be more if you are carrying more than one baby. Your extra daily calorie needs will jump to 500 calories if you breastfeed following pregnancy. It does not take much to consume an extra 300 calories. The key is to choose nutrient-rich foods that contain plenty of lean protein, complex carbohydrates, fiber, vitamins, and minerals for your extra calories. Some sensible snack ideas include:

- A red delicious apple with 2 tablespoons of chunky peanut butter (289 calories)
- One 8-ounce container of Greek-style, honey yogurt (300 calories)
- A whole-grain bagel with 1 tablespoon of cream cheese (199 calories)
- A hardboiled egg (78 calories)
- 1 cup of carrot slices (50 calories) with 4 tablespoons of light ranch dressing (131 calories)
- A 6-ounce baked potato, with skin, topped with 2 ounces of low-fat cheese, ½ cup of broccoli, and ¼ cup of salsa (300 calories)

- ½ cup tuna salad, half a piece of pita bread, lettuce, tomato, with 1 tablespoon low-fat mayo (300 calories)

Try not to skip meals, and choose nutrient-rich foods that contain plenty of lean protein (60 grams daily is ideal), fiber, vitamins, and minerals and are light on sugar, salt, and saturated and trans fats. If you are having twins or triplets, you will need to increase your calorie intake earlier; always talk to your doctor about what's right for you.

At the Doctor's or Midwife's Office

Set up your first prenatal care visit as soon as you know you are pregnant. For now through the seventh month, you'll be seeing your provider on a monthly basis (unless you are considered high risk, in which case you may have more frequent appointments). If you still haven't chosen a provider, now is the time to do so.

Your First Visit

When you go to the doctor or midwife for your first checkup, you will likely experience the following:

1. Undergo a thorough physical examination.
2. Give a urine sample (the first of many).
3. Have blood drawn for routine lab work.
4. If you haven't had a Pap smear in the last three months, your provider may also take a vaginal swab of cells scraped from your cervix for this purpose.
5. Have your pregnancy confirmed.

PRENATAL VISIT NOTES

Stats

Weight

....

Week of pregnancy

....

Fundal height

....

Blood pressure

....

Baby's heart rate

....

Tests

Test   Result

....

....

....

....

Additional Notes

....

....

....

....

Estimating Your Due Date

Most providers determine gestational age (how far along you are) from the first day of your last menstrual period (LMP). If you have a regular twenty-eight-day cycle, you can figure out your own estimated due date.

1. Take the date of your last period. _____
2. Count three months back. _____
3. Add seven days. _____
4. The resulting date _____ is your Estimated Due Date.

For example, if your last period began on September 1, you would go back through August 1 and July 1 to June 1. Then add seven days to come up with an estimated due date of June 8. An alternate method is to count 280 days (40 weeks) from the first day of your last period.

When to Contact Your Doctor or Midwife

If you experience any of the following symptoms, call your doctor or midwife immediately:

- Abdominal pain and/or cramping
- Fluid or blood leaking from the vagina
- Abnormal vaginal discharge (foul smelling, green, or yellow)
- Painful urination
- Severe headache
- Impaired vision (spots or blurring)
- Fever over 101°F
- Chills
- Excessive swelling of face and/or body

- Severe and unrelenting vomiting and/or diarrhea
- Fainting or dizziness, especially if they are accompanied by abdominal pain or bleeding (They could be symptoms of ectopic, or tubal, pregnancy, a potentially fatal condition where implantation occurs outside of the endometrial lining of the uterus, such as in the fallopian tubes.)

While a good dose of common sense should be used in contacting your doctor or midwife after hours, in most cases better safe than sorry applies. Trust your instincts. If something just doesn't feel right to you, make the call.

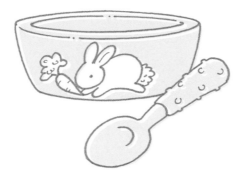

Here is a place for you to record the thoughts, feelings, and physical changes you experience during your first month of pregnancy.

Time until due date: _____

Firsts:

....

....

....

Concerns:

....

....

....

Looking forward to:

....

....

....

Questions for the doctor or midwife next month:

....

....

....

Journal

Date :   /   /

Finding Out: How did you find out you were pregnant? Was it a surprise to you or had you been trying to conceive for a while? Who was the first person you shared the news with? How did they react?

Journal

Date :   /   /

Journal

Date :   /   /

Journal

Date :   /   /

PART 3

Month Two

You've made it into month two, or weeks six through ten, of your pregnancy. By the end of this month, your baby will have outgrown her embryonic development and matured into a fetus. Your body is changing rapidly. You may start to feel pregnant now, if you didn't feel so before.

Month Two Checklist

✓ Start developing a maternity wardrobe.
✓ Make room for your baby.
✓ Create a baby-safe car environment.

Your Baby This Month

Your unborn child has now advanced from raisin to raspberry size—about ½" in length. By the end of the month, she will be about 1" long. Your baby is lengthening and straightening from the curled form she held last month. The tail she was sporting disappears around week eight, and her closed eyes start to move from the sides of her head to their permanent location. The face is further defined by a nose and jaw, and the buds of twenty tiny baby teeth are present in the gums by week ten. The palate and vocal cords also form around this time. Important organ systems are nearly completed by the end of this second month. The right and left hemispheres of your baby's brain are fully formed, and brain cell mass grows rapidly. Soft bones begin to develop, and the liver starts to manufacture red blood cells until the bone marrow can take over the job in the third trimester.

Your Body's Changes

Check off which of the following symptoms you experience this month to look back on the progress of your pregnancy and talk to your doctor or midwife about any that make you especially uncomfortable:

— Frequent urination
— Tender, larger breasts
— Increased vaginal discharge
— Occasional dizziness or faintness
— Indigestion or gas
— Headaches
— Nasal congestion and/or runny nose
— Increased saliva

On Your Mind

Now that you're feeling more symptoms of pregnancy, the reality of impending parenthood may suddenly hit home. Understanding and recognizing your emotional changes can help you better control your stress levels and mood swings.

It's easy to get stressed out over what may seem like an overwhelming amount of preparation for your new family member. Your body is already working overtime on the development of your child; try to keep your commitments and activities at a reasonable level to prevent mental and physical overload.

As you rush to get everything "just so," remember that your little one is not going to care if the crib matches the dresser, but he will feel the effects of your excess tension. Take steps to decompress when you do feel the pressure building by practicing relaxation and meditation techniques (e.g., progressive muscle relaxation, yoga with your doctor's consent), adjustments to your work or social schedule, or carving out an hour of "me" time each evening to decompress.

Eating for Two

Pregnant women are in the higher-risk category when it comes to contracting foodborne illnesses, such as listeriosis. Practice good food-safety techniques to prevent bacterial contamination of food. The U.S. government's food safety website at *www.foodsafety.gov* has more information.

Certain foods are off limits in pregnancy due to health and safety concerns. Keep this list close as a reference for when you're shopping or eating out.

- Unpasteurized milk and soft cheeses, and food made with these products.
- Unpasteurized juices and ciders.
- Raw sprouts.
- Prepared deli meats and hot dogs, unless cooked to steaming (at least 165°F).
- Raw or undercooked fish, shellfish, meat, and poultry.
- Raw or undercooked eggs or foods that contain these (e.g., eggnog, cookie dough, hollandaise sauce).
- Refrigerated pâtés, meat spreads, and smoked seafood unless cooked to steaming (at least 165°F).
- Fish high in mercury (shark, tilefish, swordfish, and king mackerel).

Steps to Keep Food Safe

Since you cannot always tell whether a food is contaminated, it is vital to take important steps to keep all of your food safe from harmful bacteria. To decrease your risk of contracting a foodborne illness, always wash your hands with hot, soapy water before and after handling foods. In addition, wash cutting boards, other work surfaces, and utensils with soap and hot water after contact with raw meat, poultry, or fish. In fact, it is best to use separate cutting boards, plates, storage containers, and utensils for raw meat and other foods. Thoroughly cooking all meat, poultry, and seafood can greatly help decrease the risk of contracting a foodborne illness. To help prevent listeria, reheat all meats purchased at the deli counter, including cured meats like salami, before eating them. Keep your raw foods separate from cooked or ready-to-eat foods so they don't contaminate them. Change sponges, dishcloths, and dishrags frequently. Always wash fruits and vegetables thoroughly with warm water before eating, and remove surface dirt with a scrub brush.

Refrigerate all of your leftovers promptly, and stay away from cooked food that has been out of the refrigerator for more than two hours. Use a thermometer to make sure that the temperature in your refrigerator is 40°F or below and that the freezer is 0°F or below to slow the growth of bacteria. The danger zone for foods is between 40°F and 140°F. Thawing meats and seafood can be a breeding ground for bacteria if they are not defrosted properly. The safest way to thaw frozen meats or seafood is in the refrigerator. Pay attention to labels on products that must be refrigerated or that have a "use by" date. Avoid dented or swollen cans, cracked jars, and loose lids that can contain bacteria. The best rule of thumb is "When in doubt, throw it out!"

At the Doctor's or Midwife's Office

If you had your preliminary appointment last month, your prenatal office visits will now start to slip into a routine. At the start of each appointment, expect to:

- Step on the scale
- Give a urine sample
- Have your blood pressure checked
- Be asked about any new or continuing pregnancy symptoms
- Have your provider feel the outside of your abdomen

Bring along that list of questions that have come up since your last visit. Write these down at the conclusion of each chapter when they come to you and your partner so they are easy to find and you won't have to rely on your memory at the office.

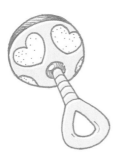

PRENATAL VISIT NOTES

Stats

Weight

....

Week of pregnancy

....

Fundal height

....

Blood pressure

....

Baby's heart rate

....

Tests

Test   Result

....

....

....

....

Additional Notes

....

....

....

....

Modifying Your Living Space

During the second month of pregnancy, start thinking about where your baby will be sleeping (or not sleeping) and playing so you can coordinate logistics and gear. If you're torn about giving up your study for a nursery (after all, she's small—how much space can she need?), think about the baby basics—crib, changing area, and dresser—plus all the inevitable stuff you're bound to acquire—swing, stuffed animals, bouncy chair, baby books, and bathtub—and the choice becomes clear.

Making Room

If a nursery isn't an option due to the size of your home or financial considerations, there are several ways to give your baby a place of her own by separating out a part of a room, including:

- Using a folding screen (or two)
- Hanging curtains from a ceiling track
- Building a wall for a more permanent partition

Nursery Safety

Evaluate the area for safety hazards. Make sure that you have:

— No peeling paint
— No dangling blind cords
— No loose flooring
— No two-piece doorstoppers (the rubber bumpers on many models can be a choking hazard)
— No decorative crib features that could potentially catch on clothing or entrap the baby
— A crib that meets federal safety standards
— A mattress that fits snugly against the crib sides

Baby Proofing

Although your home safety efforts will undoubtedly pick up steam as your child gets mobile and starts exploring her surroundings, there are some basic things you can do now to protect her in infancy and beyond. Check off the following precautions as you complete them:

Register for recalls. Take the time to fill out those registration cards for all the baby gear you receive, including your child's crib. If a safety recall of the product occurs, the manufacturer will be able to notify you. You can also register for e-mail alerts of new product recalls from the U.S. Consumer Product Safety Commission at *www.cpsc.gov*.

Ban cigarettes. You already know how dangerous it is to smoke during pregnancy, but did you know that secondhand smoke, particularly in a closed home environment, is harmful to your baby's health?

Get the lead out. Lead paint and lead solder, most frequently found in homes built before 1978, is a major hazard to small children. When ingested, it can cause central nervous system damage and developmental problems. Contact a lead inspector to test your home for the presence of lead and to advise you on abatement procedures.

Rearrange the furniture. Block off electrical cords and buy plastic protectors to seal up open outlets. Pad sharp table corners to protect your baby from injury.

Move dangerous items. Store medications, cleaning products, and plastic bags out of a child's reach.

Put the lid down. Make sure all members of the household leave the toilet seat (and lid) down. Small children are top heavy; if they peer into the toilet, they can fall in, but aren't strong enough to get out.

Evaluate your home from a baby's-eye view. Crawl around your home. Pay special attention to anything about three feet off the floor and move anything dangerous, expensive, or breakable to higher ground.

Car Safety

Cast a critical eye toward your current vehicle to make sure it meets both the practical and safety concerns of your growing family. Check to make sure your current vehicle meets the following safety standards and allows you to take suggested precautions when baby arrives. If you have not checked off the entire list, record below what remains to be done to make your car baby safe before your baby is born.

Sit back and be safe. The best place for any child is the back seat. If you have the choice, avoid pickup trucks or other vehicles that don't offer one.

Turn off the front air bag. If your new baby must ride in the front passenger seat and there is an air bag, there absolutely must be a switch that allows you to disengage the air bag on that side. If your vehicle doesn't have a switch, obtain permission to install one from the National Highway Traffic Safety Administration (NHTSA). Check with your state's motor vehicle bureau for details.

Scrutinize the side air bag (SAB). Chest and head/chest rear-seat side air bags can also pose a significant risk of injury to children, while roof-mounted head SABs are considered safe. If the vehicle has an activated rear-seat side air bag, check with the car manufacturer or the NHTSA to make sure it has been adequately tested for safe use with children. Otherwise, have it deactivated.

Choose the right seat. Make sure your baby's car seat fits properly in the vehicle and there is adequate room if you have more than one child to secure. Remember, your little one should ride in a rear-facing car seat until she reaches the top height or weight limit allowed by the seat's manufacturer (between ages 1 and 3).

Use locking seat belts, tethers, or anchors. Most vehicles built after 2002 accommodate a LATCH system (lower anchors and tethers for children) that allows you to secure the top and side tethers on a LATCH-equipped child seat to anchors built into the car interior. If your car seat or vehicle is not LATCH equipped, cars built after 1996 should have belts that work with most car seats. Always check the owner's manual of your vehicle and car seat for proper installation instructions.

Check the interior trunk release. If your car was manufactured after September 2001, it should have a release mechanism inside the trunk to prevent curious children from becoming trapped inside. Retrofitted release latches are available for cars without this feature.

Don't run hot and cold. If your car's heating and cooling system is out of commission, now is the time to get it fixed. An infant's internal thermostat is not as efficient as an adult's, and your child can quickly become overheated or chilled.

Accessorize. Car seat belts and buckles left in the sun can pose a burn hazard, so consider a car seat cover or window and windshield sun screens, which are also useful in preventing your car's interior from absorbing the sun's heat.

Other features that may be helpful but aren't absolutely essential include built-in child car seats and safety door and window locks.

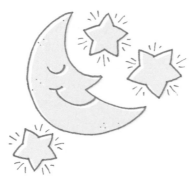

MILESTONES

Here is a place for you to record the thoughts, feelings, and physical changes you experience during your second month of pregnancy.

Time until due date: _____

Firsts:

....

....

....

Concerns:

....

....

....

Looking forward to:

....

....

....

Questions for the doctor or midwife next month:

....

....

....

Journal

Date :   /   /

Motherhood: Do you have any fears about motherhood? When you think about how your mother raised you, are there traditions, attitudes, and values you'd like to pass along to your child? How about things you'd like to do differently?

Journal

Date :   /   /

Journal

Date :   /   /

Journal

Date :   /   /

Journal

Date :   /   /

PART 4

Month Three

This is a landmark month as you finish up your first trimester! By the end of this month, your baby will grow to more than 3" in length and almost 1 ounce, about the size and heft of a roll of Life Savers. His head accounts for one-third of his total length, and his tongue, salivary glands, and taste buds have formed. You make first contact this month as you hear his heartbeat and perhaps even see him on ultrasound.

Month Three Checklist

✓ Create ways to compensate for forgetfulness.
✓ Make sleep a priority; set a new early bedtime and stick to it.

Your Baby This Month

Your baby's heart is pumping about twenty-five quarts of blood each day, and a lattice of blood vessels can be seen through his translucent skin, which is starting to develop a coat of fine downy hair called lanugo. His, or her, gender is apparent, since the external sex organs have now fully differentiated, but it will take a combination of luck and technical skill for an ultrasound operator to reveal if you have a son or daughter.

Your Body's Changes

This month, you start to sport a protruding belly, which may mean sharing your news with friends, family, and coworkers if you haven't already. Your uterus is about the size of a softball and stretches to just about your pubic bone. Two to four pounds of total weight gain is about average for the first trimester; if you've been down and out with nausea and vomiting, you may be below the curve. Weight gain will pick up in the second trimester and peak in the third, as your baby starts to fill out your womb.

While 25–35 pounds is the average suggested total weight gain for a pregnancy, your height and build will influence that number. Underweight women and women with multiple pregnancies (twins or more) will be expected to gain more; overweight women will be encouraged to gain slightly less.

If your provider hasn't mentioned a weight goal for your pregnancy, ask for your weight goal and record it here:

My Pregnancy Weight Goal: _____

Focus on the quality of food you're eating and on getting some regular exercise (cleared with your provider first).

Where the Weight Goes

Baby	7.5–8.5 pounds
Uterus	2–2.5 pounds
Placenta	1.5–2 pounds
Amniotic fluid	2 pounds
Blood	3–4 pounds
Breasts	1–2 pounds
Maternal fat and nutrient stores	4–6 pounds
Retained maternal fluids	4–8 pounds
Total	**25–35 pounds**

Although nausea and vomiting may finally be waning, constipation, gas, and occasional heartburn may take over as the gastrointestinal pests of the second trimester.

Constipation can be caused by an increase in progesterone, which can act to slow down the digestive system. Later in the pregnancy, pressure on the intestines caused by your growing uterus adds to the problem. Iron supplements or prenatal vitamins with added iron can also cause constipation, so talking to your provider about the possibility of a dosage adjustment or an extended release formula may be in order. An increase in dietary fiber, plenty of water intake, and exercise as approved by your healthcare provider may also help to get things going again. Be sure to consult your doctor before taking any stool softeners or laxatives.

Other pregnancy symptoms that may continue or begin this month include the following. Check off symptoms you experience this month and talk to your doctor or midwife about any that make you especially uncomfortable:

— Fatigue
— Frequent urination
— Tender breasts
— Occasional dizziness or faintness
— Headaches
— Nasal congestion and/or runny nose
— Increased saliva
— Nausea

On Your Mind

Like any mom-to-be, you've got a lot on your mind. That alone may have you forgetting what used to be second nature, and misplacing things. Pregnancy hormones, sleep deprivation, and stress have all been suggested as possible culprits.

Whatever the cause, forgetting appointments and misplacing things can leave you feeling muddled and helpless. To cope with forgetfulness, try the following:

- Writing notes and keeping lists
- Sticking to a routine (e.g., car keys always go into a basket by the door)
- Living by a written or electronic organizer
- Requesting a twenty-four-hour advance phone call reminder when you schedule appointments

Eating for Two

Swapping ingredients in your recipes for leaner ones can healthy-up your meals. Small changes within a recipe can make big differences in the nutritional outcome. You may need to use less of an ingredient, substitute an ingredient, add a new ingredient, or completely leave something out. It will take some trial and error to get your recipes to your liking, but the extra effort will be well worth it.

Take a look at your recipes before you get started, and think about what individual ingredients may contribute to a dish that's higher in fat, cholesterol, calories, or sodium. Decide which ingredients can be substituted or reduced as well as added for additional nutritional value. Adding shredded carrots or zucchini to your lasagna, for example, can add a load of extra vitamins, minerals, and fiber to your dish. Make changes to your recipes gradually by changing one or two ingredients at a time each time you make it.

Use some of these substitutions to cut fat and calories while cooking or baking:

- Use fat-free or low-fat milk instead of whole milk.
- Use low-fat yogurt, ½ cup cottage cheese blended with 1½ teaspoons lemon juice, or light or fat-free sour cream instead of regular sour cream.

- Use evaporated fat-free milk or fat-free half-and-half instead of cream.
- Use 3 tablespoons cocoa powder plus 1 tablespoon oil instead of 1 ounce unsweetened baking chocolate.
- Use low-fat cottage cheese or low-fat or nonfat ricotta cheese instead of regular ricotta cheese.
- Use chocolate sauce instead of fudge sauce.
- Use nonfat or low-fat plain yogurt or reduced-fat mayonnaise instead of regular mayonnaise.
- Use puréed fruits such as applesauce to replace anywhere from a third to half of the fat in recipes.
- For pies and other desserts, use a graham-cracker-crumb crust instead of a higher-fat pastry shell.
- Use puréed cooked vegetables instead of cream, egg yolks, or roux to thicken sauces and soups.

Vegetarian and Vegan Pregnancy Nutrition

Vegetarian and vegan moms-to-be can have perfectly safe and healthy pregnancies without giving up their lifestyles. You'll just need to carefully monitor some key nutrients. Eating a variety of foods including fruits, vegetables, plenty of leafy greens, whole-grain products, beans, nuts, and seeds virtually ensures that you'll meet most of your nutrient needs.

One nutrient that vegetarians and vegans are often asked about is protein. Although many foods provide some protein, the dried bean family is an especially good way to get protein. From vegetarian baked beans to chili (*sin carne*—without meat) to lentil soup, it's easy to add beans to your diet. Soy products such as tofu, tempeh, soymilk, textured vegetable protein (TVP), and edamame are also high in protein. Don't forget other foods including whole grains, nuts, nut butters, vegetables, potatoes, and seeds (pumpkin, sesame, sunflower, etc.) that are also great ways to add to your protein totals.

Iron and zinc needs are increased in a vegetarian and vegan diet because they are not absorbed as easily from beans and grains. There are some tricks to increase your absorption of these minerals. Including a food with vitamin C (citrus, tomatoes, cabbage, or broccoli, for instance) at most meals can markedly boost iron and zinc absorption. Good sources of iron and zinc for vegans include enriched breakfast cereals, wheat germ, soy products, dried beans, pumpkin and sunflower seeds, and dark chocolate.

Calcium and vitamin D are important for strong bones. Contrary to what you may have been told, you don't need to have a cow-milk mustache in order to get enough of these nutrients. Some vegetarian and vegan foods are fortified with calcium and vitamin D. Check labels of soymilk and other plant milks to make sure they have vitamin D and calcium added to them. Calcium is also found in foods like dark leafy greens, tofu set with calcium salts, and dried figs. Vitamin D can also be produced by your skin when you're out in the sun. Vegan vitamin D supplements are another way to meet your vitamin D needs. And, of course, exercise is a key requirement for building strong bones.

Vitamin B_{12} cannot be reliably obtained from unfortified vegan foods, but there are vegan foods that are fortified with this important vitamin. Fortified foods include some brands of breakfast cereals, nutritional yeast, plant-based milks, and mock meats. If you're not sure whether or not you're getting enough vitamin B_{12} from fortified foods, a vitamin B_{12} supplement is a wise idea.

Fish and fish oils are often promoted as sources of omega-3 fatty acids. Vegetarians and vegans have other options. You can get omega-3s from flaxseeds, flax oil, walnuts, hempseeds, and other foods. There are even vegan versions of the omega-3 fatty acids found in fish oil—DHA and EPA.

By making smart food choices, it's easy to eat a healthy vegetarian or vegan diet—one that's good for you, for your baby-to-be, and for the planet.

At the Doctor's or Midwife's Office

This month, your provider may:

- Order an ultrasound to see your baby
- Start estimating the size of your baby by counting the centimeters from your pubic bone to the tip of your fundus—the top of the uterus (some practitioners do not take the fundal height until after week twelve or even week twenty)
- Offer to take a pregnancy-associated plasma protein-A (PAPP-A) and human chorionic gonadotropic (hCG) blood test to screen for Down syndrome and trisomy 18
- Check for the fetal heartbeat using a small ultrasound device called a Doppler or Doptone

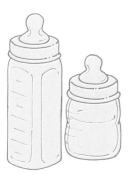

PRENATAL VISIT NOTES

Stats

Weight
....

Week of pregnancy
....

Fundal height
....

Blood pressure
....

Baby's heart rate
....

Tests

Test   Result

....

....

....

....

Additional Notes

....

....

....

....

MILESTONES

Here is a place for you to record the thoughts, feelings, and physical changes you experience during your third month of pregnancy.

Time until due date: _____

Firsts:

....

....

....

Concerns:

....

....

....

Looking forward to:

....

....

....

Questions for the doctor or midwife next month:

....

....

....

Journal

Date :   /   /

Fatherhood: How is your baby's daddy coping with the idea of parenthood? What kind of dad do you think he will be? What traits do you hope your child inherits from him?

Journal

Date :   /   /

Journal

Date :   /   /

Journal

Date :   /   /

PART 5

Month Four

Welcome to the second trimester, or what many women consider the fun part. Your energy is up, and your meals are staying down. You and your baby are headed into a period of rapid growth now, so hang on and enjoy the ride.

Month Four Checklist

✓ Treat yourself to a special day out.
✓ Begin keeping a food log.
✓ If you don't have one, shop for a crib that meets current safety standards.
✓ Create a prenatal exercise routine.

Your Baby This Month

Snoozing, stretching, swallowing, and even thumb sucking, your baby is busy this month as she tests out her new reflexes and abilities. She is losing her top-heavy look as her height starts to catch up to her head size. By the end of this month, she will measure about 6"–8" in length and weigh approximately 6 ounces.

Your Body's Changes

If you weren't showing last month, chances are you will have a definite pregnant profile by the end of this month. Your uterus is about the size of a head of cabbage, and its top lies just below your belly button.

Your appetite may start to pick up this month, especially if you've been too sick to enjoy a good meal until now. About 60 percent of your total pregnancy weight (about 11–15 pounds) will be gained in this trimester.

Other symptoms of second-trimester pregnancy you may start or continue to experience this month include the following. Check off those that you are experiencing so that you may discuss relief with your doctor:

— Hemorrhoids
— Nausea
— Fatigue
— Frequent urination
— Tender and/or swollen breasts
— Bleeding gums
— Excess mucus and saliva
— Increase in vaginal discharge
— Mild shortness of breath
— Lightheadedness or dizziness
— Gas and/or constipation
— Skin and hair changes
— Feeling warm or easily overheated

On Your Mind

You're hitting your stride as the wooziness and uncertainties of the first three months fade away, and the discomforts of late pregnancy still lie relatively far ahead.

Feeling better and having more energy, you may be ready to conquer the world (or at least the nursery). For many women, the starter's pistol on motherhood goes off right when they feel baby's first pokes and prods. The palpable presence of your child may trigger a series of mothering emotions—protectiveness, nurturing, nesting—and complete and total impatience with anyone who poses a potential threat to the well-being of you and your child.

Eating for Two

Heartburn may start to become a persistent problem as your uterus crowds your stomach and the smooth muscles of your digestive tract remain relaxed from the hormone progesterone. Some tips for putting out the fire include:

- Avoid greasy, fatty, and spicy foods.
- Stay away from alcohol and caffeinated drinks (e.g., cola, tea, coffee); these may relax the valve between the stomach and the esophagus and exacerbate heartburn.
- Eat smaller, more frequent meals instead of three large ones.
- Drink plenty of water between meals to reduce stomach acid.
- Don't eat just before you go to bed or lay down to rest.
- Pile a few extra pillows on the bed to assist gravity in easing heartburn while you sleep.

Another option you have is to keep a food diary to try to determine what your heartburn triggers are to avoid them in the future.

At the Doctor's or Midwife's Office

If you didn't get to listen to your baby's heartbeat last month, you'll likely get your chance with this visit. Women who have chosen to take an alpha-fetoprotein (AFP) test will have their blood drawn sometime between weeks sixteen and eighteen. The AFP is typically given at sixteen to eighteen weeks, and it tests for the possibility of neural tube defects and/or chromosomal abnormalities.

PRENATAL VISIT NOTES

Stats

Weight

Week of pregnancy

Fundal height

Blood pressure

Baby's heart rate

Tests

Test

Result

Additional Notes

Movement!

If this is your second or third child, you may already recognize the familiar sensation of your baby's body flexing in your womb. For moms in their debut pregnancy with somewhat less stretchy accommodations, the first movements—known as quickening—may not be felt quite as early. By week nineteen, most women have felt that distinctive first flutter.

So what does it feel like? Record what those first baby movements felt like for you.

....

....

....

Once your baby starts moving regularly, the sensation becomes second nature. When you begin to feel your baby moving regularly, try to record how many movements you feel within a few hours to get an idea of your baby's average number of movements per hour.

Hour One   _____
Hour Two   _____
Hour Three   _____

On average, you should feel four or more movements each hour from your passenger. Three or fewer movements or a sudden decrease in fetal activity could be a sign of fetal distress, so if you notice either, call your provider as soon as possible to follow up.

Exercise

Don't avoid the gym, pool, or other favorite fitness hangouts just because you're pregnant. Exercise will make you feel better, and it can tone muscles that will be getting a workout in labor and delivery (be sure, though, to check with your healthcare provider before beginning an exercise routine). For women in regular pregnancies (i.e., not high risk), thirty minutes of moderate exercise daily is ideal. Consider the benefits a regular workout may provide:

- **Keep energy up.** Stretching and moving daily will boost your energy level.
- **Relax.** Exercise can help calm your mind.
- **Get postpartum weight down.** It will be easier to work off your pregnancy weight after the birth if you already have a regular routine.
- **Ease your aches and pains.** Exercise that promotes strength and flexibility can prevent or diminish lower back pain, muscle aches, and other complaints of pregnancy.
- **Foster a positive mental attitude.** Feeling fit may improve your self-image.

It's best to avoid exercises that can cause you to become overheated or that involve bouncing, jarring, sudden changes in direction, lifting, or a risk of falling. Here are some generally safe pregnancy exercise ideas:

Golf (sans cart)	Stretching exercises with a pregnancy ball
Hiking	Swimming
Light weight lifting	Walking
Stair climbing	Water aerobics
Stationary biking	Yoga

Spreading the Word

Here are some ideas for sharing the news with family and friends:

- Give them an ultrasound picture (or a photocopy of one).
- Send out birthday invitations for the estimated due date.
- Take out a "Help Wanted: Grandparents" advertisement in their local classifieds and point them to it.
- Invite them to dinner (at home or out) and serve a frosting-inscribed "It's a Boy/Girl/Baby," "Congratulations Auntie," or "We're Pregnant" cake for dessert.
- Ask them to go shopping with you and take them to your four-month doctor's or midwife's appointment instead.
- If this isn't your first, let your kids spread the news in their own special way.
- The old standby—"Guess what?"—works well, too.

Working Through Pregnancy

Make sure that your employer hears about your pregnancy from you, and not around the water cooler, first. Accompany the news with your tentative schedule for maternity leave so your manager can plan accordingly.

If this is your first child, it can be hard to fully assess the new career direction you're taking. But there are probably some basic decisions you can make with a degree of certainty. For example, late shifts and double-overtime may be out of the picture for you now.

You should also ask questions to determine whether your company is even worth sticking with through your pregnancy and beyond. Comment in the spaces below to see how your company stacks up in the family friendly category.

Flexibility: Does the company have written policies on options like flex time, job sharing, and telecommuting?

....

....

....

Lactation facilities: Are there appropriate, comfortable areas dedicated to breastfeeding or breast milk pumping? If not, is your employer willing to provide an appropriate, private space?

....

....

....

Paid paternity leave: Are dads given time off for a new baby with pay, or at least without prejudice? If a policy is in place, is it used successfully?

....

....

....

On-site child care or child care assistance: If your workplace doesn't have on-site or sponsored child care, does it offer enrollment in a tax-free flexible spending account that allows you to save up to $5,000 tax free to pay child care expenses?

....

....

....

Time-saving perks: These may run the gamut from on-site dry cleaning and retail services to employee concierge services that can run small errands for you.

....

....

....

Value placed on education: Corporate-sponsored scholarships for children of employees, tuition assistance, and mentorship programs with local schools are a few ways a company may express the value of education.

....

....

....

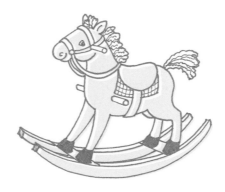

CAREER FUTURE SHEET

Ask yourself the following questions to assess the career direction you may want to take and decide what are feasible goals for your job future.

Do you want to move into a supervisory position at your next review? Do you see your company promoting people who work excessive overtime? If so, are you capable of committing to working extra hours after your baby is born?

....
....
....

Will you require an extremely or moderately flexible job?

....
....
....

Is your partner's job flexible enough to allow your job to be less so?

....
....
....

Do you intend to advance in your current career and become or remain the primary earner in your family, or will your partner take on that role?

....
....
....

Are you a single parent who will be relying on your own income after your baby is born?

....

....

....

....

Do you have options for affordable child care for when your baby is born? How does this affect your postpartum working schedule?

....

....

....

....

Is your job adaptable so that you can work from home? If not, would you like a job that is?

....

....

....

....

....

After completing the previous questionnaire, you can use your answers to create career goals based on what job characteristics you will be looking for once your child is born.

Career/Lifestyle Goal

How to Achieve My Goal

Have afternoons off

Become a part-time speech therapist instead of a full-time speech therapist.

....

....

....

....

....

....

....

....

....

....

....

....

....

....

....

....

....

....

....

....

....

....

....

....

....

....

Maternity Leave

It's a good idea to put all maternity leave plans in writing for your supervisor and appropriate managers and to make an extra copy for placement in your personnel file.

Lay the groundwork for your maternity leave so there won't be too many questions or crises in your absence. If appropriate for your position, delegate some tasks to coworkers and arrange coverage by others.

Check and double-check that all appropriate benefits paperwork has been filled out, signed off, and sent in well in advance of your planned departure. Maternity leave should be a low-stress time, not one that requires twice-weekly contact with human resources to find out the status of your disability claim.

So just how much, or how little, maternity leave should you take? Certainly the benefits your company provides will play a major factor in your decision. Factors to consider include:

Flexibility: Does the company have written policies on options like flex time, job sharing, and telecommuting?

....

....

....

....

....

....

....

Money: How much time off can you afford if your maternity benefits are minimal or nonexistent? Don't forget to factor any money you'll be saving—such as dry-cleaning bills, lunches out, and transportation expenses—into your equation.

....

....

....

....

....

....

....

Management: Even though you may be legally within your rights, in some organizations an extended maternity leave may be frowned upon by those above you. What might management think, and more important, what kind of priority do you place on their disapproval?

....

....

....

....

....

....

....

Morale: Are your coworkers and/or subordinates happy and motivated or disillusioned and bitter? Employees who work as a team and feel invested in their workplace are more likely to rise to the challenge in your absence.

....

....

....

....

....

....

....

Malleability: Does it have to be all or nothing? Think about offering some creative proposals for extending your leave, such as a reduced part-time schedule or telecommuting.

....

....

....

....

....

....

....

Full Time at Home

Finally, for the woman who wants it all and wants it close to home, consider the possibility of forging your own family-friendly path. Many occupations lend themselves to home-based work, such as:

- Writing
- Income tax preparation
- Desktop publishing
- Web design
- Refinishing antiques
- Creating crafts for retail
- Sewing
- Painting

Additional ideas for a home-based business:

....

....

....

....

....

....

....

....

....

....

....

MATERNITY LEAVE PLANNER

Estimated due date:
....

Employer insurance benefits offered:
....

....

....

Total leave requested:
....

Amount of paid time off:
....

Amount of unpaid time off:
....

Estimated cost of unpaid time off:
....

Replacement arrangement (temporary help, coworker replacement, etc.):
....

....

....

....

Responsibilities to take care of before leave:
....

....

....

....

....

Here is a place for you to record the thoughts, feelings, and physical changes you experience during your fourth month of pregnancy.

Time until due date: _____

Firsts:

....

....

....

Concerns:

....

....

....

Looking forward to:

....

....

....

Questions for the doctor or midwife next month:

....

....

....

Journal

Date :   /   /

Changing Habits: What are some of the things you've had to give up or change with your pregnancy? Has it been hard? Do you plan to go back to your prepregnancy ways once baby arrives?

Journal

Date :   /   /

Journal

Date :   /   /

Journal

Date :   /   /

Journal

Date :   /   /

PART 6

Month Five

This month, you're still enjoying the relative comfort level of the second trimester, but your energy and initiative may be slightly dampened by the dwindling quality of your sleep. Sleep deprivation can also contribute to mental fuzziness and emotional edginess. Now's the time to value and prioritize time spent sleeping.

Month Five Checklist

✓ Plan a special night out with your partner.
✓ Choose a method of childbirth instruction.
✓ Tour childbirth centers.

Your Baby This Month

At 10"–12" long and around 1 pound in weight, your baby is about the size of a football. He is starting to bulk up a bit as he accumulates deposits of brown fat under his skin. This insulation will help regulate his body temperature in the outside world. He's using his bulk to make his presence known; if you weren't feeling him last month you likely are now.

Your baby is now covered in a white oily substance known as vernix caseosa, a sort of full-body fetal ChapStick that keeps his fluid-soaked skin from peeling and protects against infection.

Your Body's Changes

As your baby grows, your muscles and ligaments stretch to support this new weight. The result may be a new set of aches and pains as your body adjusts to the load.

The skin of your belly is stretching, tightening, and itching like crazy. A good moisturizing cream can relieve the itching and keep your skin hydrated, although it won't prevent or eliminate striae gravidarum, or stretch marks.

The band of ligaments supporting your uterus is carrying an increasingly heavy load. You may start to feel occasional discomfort in your lower abdomen, inner thighs, and hips called round ligament pain. Pelvic tilt exercises are useful for keeping pelvic muscles toned and relieving pain. To perform the pelvic tilt:

1. Kneel on all fours on the floor.
2. Keeping your head aligned with your spine, pull in your abdomen, tighten your buttocks, and tilt your pelvis forward. Your back will naturally arch up.
3. Hold the position for three seconds, then relax. (Remember to keep your back straight in this neutral position.)
4. Repeat the tilt three to five times, eventually working up to ten repetitions.

The root of all things uncomfortable—pregnancy hormones—are also contributing to lower back pain you may be experiencing. Progesterone and relaxin—the hormone responsible for softening your pelvic ligaments for delivery—are also loosening up your lower back ligaments and disks, and combined with the weight of your growing belly your back is feeling the strain.

If your abdominal and/or back pains are severe or accompanied by any of the following, call your healthcare provider immediately:

- Fever
- Vomiting
- Vaginal bleeding
- Leg numbness

Most minor back pain of pregnancy is completely normal, but in severe cases it can be a sign of preterm labor, kidney infection, or other medical problems.

To help you ease your aches and pains:

Stand tall. Try to keep your center of gravity in your spine and pelvis rather than out in your belly, which can give you a swayback.

Sit up straight. Use good posture when you're sitting as well and choose a chair with good lower back support. You can purchase a special ergonomic support pad for your chair back, but a small pillow may do the trick just as easily.

Avoid twists and turns. With everything so loose, a sudden move as simple as quickly turning at the waist to get out of bed may strain your back. Use your arms as support for a slow takeoff when rising from a chair.

Practice your pickups. If you have small children who still need to be lifted occasionally, it's essential to use good form. To avoid injury, bend and use your leg muscles to lift things rather than bending from the waist and lifting with your back.

Warm up. A warm pad on your back, hips, or other sore spots may help relieve pain.

Wear sensible shoes. Avoid high heels! They will place further stress on your spine.

Rest your feet. Use a low stool or step to rest your feet when sitting. If you must stand for long periods, alternate resting each foot on a step.

Massage. You now have a medical excuse to indulge in a regular back rub from your significant other. A licensed massage therapist who is experienced in prenatal massage may also be helpful.

Fluff and stuff. Sleep on your side with a pillow placed between your legs. This will align your spine and improve your sleeping posture. A full-sized body pillow or beanbag may help support your back and belly as well.

Exercise. Stretching and flexibility exercises may help.

Symptoms you may start or continue to experience this month include the following. Check off any that you are experiencing so that you may ask your doctor about relief and to track the progress of your pregnancy.

— Hot flashes
— Nausea
— Fatigue
— Frequent urination
— Tender and/or swollen breasts
— Bleeding gums
— Excess mucus and saliva
— Increase in vaginal discharge
— Mild shortness of breath
— Lightheadedness or dizziness
— Headaches
— Gas
— Heartburn
— Constipation
— Skin and hair changes

On Your Mind

If family and friends are getting your ire up, it may be a sign that you are feeling overwhelmed and undersupported. Take a look at what's really getting to you. Sit down and tell your partner what you're feeling and work out some strategies for easing the burden together. It may help to write down what you are having difficulty dealing with, then work with your partner to create a solution.

Challenge	Solution
....	....
....	....
....	....
....	....
....	....
....	....
....	....
....	....
....	....
....	....
....	....
....	....
....	....

Step back and take stock. Are you making work, and stress, for yourself through self-imposed deadlines? Look at your to-do list in terms of small tasks rather than an all-or-nothing prospect. Prioritize what's there and dare to cross off a few things that just aren't that important right now.

Old To-Do List	Newly Prioritized and Shortened To-Do List
....	....
....	....
....	....
....	....
....	....
....	....
....	....
....	....
....	....
....	....

Eating for Two

Women tend to crave sweet foods more during their second trimester than at any other time in their pregnancy. A sweet tooth for healthy foods, like fruit, doesn't tend to be a problem. But when you have a serious hankering for high-sugar, high-calorie foods, it's important to curb the cravings with some simple strategies:

- **Never skip meals.** That includes breakfast. Skipping meals can increase cravings later in the day.
- **Indulge in moderation.** Treat yourself to a donut hole instead of the whole donut, or a single scoop of ice cream instead of the sundae.
- **Make smart substitutions.** Choose a fruit sorbet instead of a double-fudge sundae, or a whole-wheat bagel with fresh sliced berries, and get all the sweetness without all the added calories.
- **Stay active.** Regular exercise, even as simple as daily walks, can help control cravings.

Craving Fast Food

How many times have you been out running around—or home but not in the mood to do any cooking—and decided to stop at the first fast-food place you saw? Fast foods are more popular than ever before, and many now offer a variety of healthy menu alternatives. Still, frequenting fast-food places can lead to a higher intake of fat, calories, sodium, saturated fat, and cholesterol. It can also cut into your chances of getting in all the food groups you need each day, including fruits, vegetables, dairy, and whole grains. Some pregnant women may lose their taste altogether for that fast-food burger, while others may begin to crave them.

When choosing your fast-food entrée, choose smaller burgers without the cheese, bacon, mayonnaise, and special sauces. All these toppers add more saturated fat and cholesterol to your meal, not to mention calories. Use lower-fat toppings such as ketchup, mustard, barbecue sauces, lettuce, tomatoes, and pickles. Better yet, go for the grilled chicken breast or a sensible salad. If you choose to eat chicken or fish, stay away from the deep-fried versions, which will be high in fat and calories. A grilled, roasted, or broiled piece of chicken or fish is the healthiest choice.

Toppings can add up quickly, as follows:

- One packet of mayonnaise can have as much as 95 calories and 10 grams of fat.
- One packet of tartar sauce can add as much as 160 calories and 17 grams of fat to your fish sandwich.
- A 2-ounce packet of ranch dressing can have as much as 290 calories and 30 grams of fat.
- Just one slice of American cheese can add 50 calories and 5 grams of fat.

Subs can make for a healthy, low-fat sandwich when prepared on whole-grain bread and topped with mustard, vegetable oil, and/or low-fat cheese. Go for the cooked turkey or chicken breast instead of the higher-fat processed meats such as salami or bologna. Load up your sub with vegetables such as lettuce, tomato, onions, and peppers. Wraps are also a good choice. Again, beware of the added cheese, dressings, and sauces that can turn a simple sub into a high-fat and high-calorie nightmare. Ask for half the cheese, and ask for the dressing and sauce on the side so you can choose a lower-fat or fat-free version.

Not sure how your favorite fast-food menus rate? Most fast-food restaurants have websites that post nutritional information on their foods. Check them out before you head off to the drive-through!

At the Doctor's or Midwife's Office

Beyond the usual weigh and measure routine, your doctor or midwife may administer an oral glucose tolerance test (OGTT) at the end of the month (between weeks twenty-four and twenty-eight). If your doctor or midwife hasn't discussed counting fetal movements before, he or she may mention it now.

PRENATAL VISIT NOTES

Stats

Weight
....

Week of pregnancy
....

Fundal height
....

Blood pressure
....

Baby's heart rate
....

Tests

Test   Result

....

....

....

....

Additional Notes

....

....

....

....

Childbirth Classes

Now's a good time to start gathering information on childbirth classes from your local hospital or birthing center to give you and your partner time to decide which class is right for you. Pick a class date that falls in your third trimester so the information will still be fresh in your mind once the big day arrives. While hospital policy will dictate a lot of what's covered in prepared childbirth classes, here's a general idea of what you will experience:

- **Commiseration:** You'll interact with other pregnant couples and demonstrate that misery (and joy) truly does love company.
- **Reality:** Through lecture and (in many cases) actual video footage, you'll get the full scoop on what really goes on in labor and delivery.
- **Guided tour:** If your class is at the birthing center or hospital, you will probably get a tour of the facilities and some basic instructions on when and where to show up when labor hits.
- **Teamwork:** Your husband, partner, or labor coach will learn more about his or her role in this process, and you may even be given homework to try out techniques at home.
- **After-birth instruction:** Many classes offer valuable information on breastfeeding basics and baby care. Don't be surprised if the instructor brings in a bag full of baby dolls for practice.
- **Seasoned support:** Most prepared childbirth classes will be conducted by a trained childbirth educator.
- **Paperwork:** A lot of literature, brochures, pamphlets, handouts, forms, photocopies, and leaflets will come your way. Bring a bag.

Following are some of the most popular childbirth educational offerings for you to consider as you research your options.

Lamaze

While rhythmic breathing exercises are stressed for each stage of labor in Lamaze, helpful laboring and birth positions, relaxation techniques, and pain management are also covered. In addition to massage, water therapy, and hot and cold compresses, you're taught how to focus on a picture or object to diminish your discomfort.

Lamaze also stresses the empowerment of the mother-to-be and her right to the birth experience and environment she wants.

Bradley Method

Denver obstetrician Robert Bradley, MD, was a big advocate of fathers helping their partners through the birth process. Bradley Method classes teach couples how to relax and breathe deeply, but the emphasis is on doing what comes naturally—such as father as coach, proper nutrition during pregnancy, and knowing all the options beforehand. They also emphasize the natural in natural childbirth, suggesting that pain medication be used as a last resort rather than a front-line tool.

HypnoBirthing

British doctor and natural childbirth pioneer Grantly Dick-Read, who authored the classic *Childbirth Without Fear*, is the inspiration behind HypnoBirthing education. Dr. Dick-Read believed that a woman's labor pains were magnified by her fear and anxieties. HypnoBirthing emphasizes slow abdominal breathing and other relaxation techniques that teach you how to focus on the feelings and signals your body sends during labor.

CHILDBIRTH CLASS FOLLOW-UP SHEET

If you are still confused about different types of childbirth classes, call your hospital or birthing center and ask for printed schedules and descriptions of upcoming classes. Once you get a basic feel for what is offered, you can call with follow-up questions. Use the template below to gain as much information as you can.

What are the instructor's credentials and training?

....

What methods are taught in the class?

....

What is the typical class size?

....

What does the curriculum consist of?

....

How much does enrollment cost?

....

Are there additional costs beyond the enrollment fee, such as for study materials or learning aids?

....

Are there couples that can be contacted as references?

....

....

....

Once you have chosen which class best suits your needs and those of your partner, record any information about the class here.

Class starting date:
....

Class meeting times:
....

Class instructor:
....

Address of class:
....

Phone number of facility:
....

Additional notes:
....

....

....

When you begin taking labor classes later in your pregnancy, use this space to record notes from class. As you approach the time of labor, you can check back and review the helpful tips and techniques that you learned in childbirth class.

....

....

....

....

....

....

....

....

Touring the Hospital/Birthing Center

Even if you don't choose a childbirth class sponsored by the facility at which you'll be giving birth, you should try to arrange a tour. On the tour, you can:

- Find out where you must park when you and your partner arrive at the center.
- Get a sneak peek of the labor and birthing rooms.
- Get a feel for the staff's attitude and level of friendliness and approachability.
- Tour the nursery and maternity ward.
- Observe newborn care.
- Acquaint yourself with hospital/center policy and procedures.

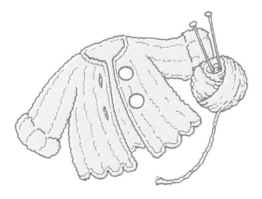

Here is a place for you to record the thoughts, feelings, and physical changes you experience during your fifth month of pregnancy.

Time until due date: _____

Firsts:

....

....

....

Concerns:

....

....

....

Looking forward to:

....

....

....

Questions for the doctor or midwife next month:

....

....

....

Journal

Date :   /   /

War Stories: What kind of advice have other mothers been offering—both wanted and unwanted? Have you heard anything that scared you? Offended you? Made you smile?

Journal

Date :   /   /

Journal

Date :　　　/　　　/

Journal

Date :   /   /

Journal

Date : / /

Journal

Date :   /   /

PART 7

Month Six

At six months, you may feel as though you'll be pregnant forever, but the final trimester will come and go before you know it. Take some time this month to savor pregnancy and treat yourself to some of the indulgences that only a mother-to-be can pull off.

Month Six Checklist

✓ Take a day off and pamper yourself.
✓ Start putting together your birth plan.
✓ Think about who you want in the delivery room.
✓ Begin listing baby names.

Your Baby This Month

Feeling a rhythmic lurch in your abdomen? Your little girl probably has the hiccups, a common phenomenon thought to be brought on by drinking and/or breathing amniotic fluid. They'll go away on their own, eventually.

The once-transparent skin of your baby is starting to thicken, and sweat glands are developing below the skin surface. She's over a foot long now, and by the end of the month she may weigh up to 2 pounds.

Your Body's Changes

Your uterus extends well above your navel now. You may actually be seeing fetal movement across your abdomen as your baby gets comfortable in her shrinking living space. You will also notice that your feet have begun to swell. This is a result of the dramatic increase in blood volume you've experienced, which is feeding excess fluids to surrounding tissues, resulting in edema (or water retention). To make matters worse, the weight of your uterus is requiring the veins in your legs to work double time to pump all that extra blood back to your heart. Estrogen also increases the amount of fluid your tissues absorb.

The result of all this is puffy and sometimes aching feet. Putting your feet up when you can, wearing comfortable low-heeled shoes, and soaking your feet in cool water are all good ways to ease the discomfort. Special compression stockings, available at medical supply stores, may also be helpful.

If you experience sudden and severe swelling of the face and hands, call your doctor or midwife immediately. It may be a sign of preeclampsia, also called toxemia, a condition that is potentially hazardous to both you and your baby. Other signs of preeclampsia include:

- High blood pressure
- Headaches
- Visual disturbances
- Sudden excessive weight gain
- Protein in the urine

Symptoms on the menu yet again this month include the following. Check off any that you are experiencing so that you can ask your doctor or midwife about them and to track the progress of your pregnancy:

— Nausea
— Fatigue
— Frequent urination
— Tender and/or swollen breasts

— Bleeding gums
— Excess mucus and saliva
— Increase in vaginal discharge
— Mild shortness of breath
— Lightheadedness or dizziness
— Headaches
— Forgetfulness
— Gas
— Heartburn
— Constipation
— Skin and hair changes
— Round ligament pain or soreness
— Lower back aches
— Mild swelling of legs, feet, and hands
— Leg cramps

On Your Mind

As you sidle up to the third trimester starting line, try to take advantage of these final days of relative comfort and sit back and savor your pregnancy. Try each of these ways to pamper yourself:

• Splurge for a day-spa treatment.
• Spend a lazy afternoon curled up with a good book.
• Enjoy a nice, relaxing soak in the tub.
• Take a scenic weekend drive with no deadlines or particular destination.
• Use the valet service to park instead of hiking from the lot.
• Order healthy carry-out fare from your favorite restaurant.

Eating for Two

During pregnancy, your body's water needs expand significantly to support amniotic fluid production and increased blood volume. You should be drinking eight to twelve 8-ounce glasses of water per day. Try keeping a bottle of water on your desk, in the car, and in other handy places as a good reminder to sip throughout the day. And keep in mind that your fluid needs may increase during hot weather, when exercising, or if you are sick with fever, vomiting, or diarrhea.

In addition to regular drinking water, other noncaffeinated beverages such as sparkling water, seltzer, vegetable juice, milk, and fruit juice can also contribute toward your daily hydration goals. Be mindful of the extra calories in fruit juice.

Always steer clear of alcohol and herbal-based beverages and energy drinks. And drink coffee, tea, and soft drinks in moderation or eliminate them completely from your pregnancy diet, as they contain caffeine.

Fitting in Fluids

Like everything else, drinking water should be part of your healthy lifestyle—you should make it a habit. Make a commitment today to start drinking water on a regular basis. You should be in the habit before you even become pregnant. You should start out with a moderate goal and work your way up. It may help to start a water diary on a calendar to keep track of your current intake and your progress. If you need help increasing your water intake, follow some of these helpful tips:

- At work or at home, take water breaks instead of coffee breaks.
- Keep a bottle of water at your desk, on your counter at home, or in your car when traveling so you have it available to sip throughout the day.

- Get in the habit of drinking a glass of water before and with meals and snacks. Besides helping you to stay hydrated, it can help take the edge off of your appetite.
- Use a straw to drink your water. Believe it or not, using a straw can help you drink faster and make a glass of water seem a little more manageable.
- Drink water instead of snacking while watching television or reading a book.
- Keep a 2-quart container of water in the refrigerator, and make it your goal to drink it all by the end of the day. This also gives you a constant supply of good, cold water.

What about Caffeine?

The risk of caffeine intake during pregnancy is a controversial issue. Still, most experts agree that you should cut back on your caffeine consumption while trying to conceive and while you are pregnant. That doesn't mean you have to completely cut out caffeine, but you should cut down. Most research shows that it is safe to drink coffee or other caffeinated beverages during pregnancy as long as you consume fewer than three cups, or about 300 mg, of caffeine per day (per the American Dietetic Association). Consumption of more than 300 mg per day has been associated with a possible decrease in fertility and an increase risk of miscarriage or low birth-weight babies.

Caffeine acts as a mild stimulant to the central nervous system and also has a diuretic effect, which increases water loss from the body through urination. Neither of these effects is favorable during pregnancy or even for good health in general. Caffeine can also decrease the amount of calcium your body absorbs and can increase loss of calcium through the urine. This effect of caffeine becomes more prominent if dietary calcium intake is already inadequate. Many over-the-counter pain relievers, cold medications, allergy medications, and diet pills contain as much caffeine as a cup or two of coffee, so read labels carefully. When purchasing over-the-counter medications, ask the pharmacist which are best. Be sure to mention that you are pregnant or trying to cut down on your caffeine intake.

While many doctors recommend cutting back on caffeine, others recommend cutting it out of your diet completely, especially if you are in a high-risk category. Some doctors may recommend cutting out caffeine completely during the first trimester and then restricting amounts during the remainder of the pregnancy. Talk with your doctor about your best options. Decaffeinated beverages are fine, but be sure they are not crowding out more nutritious beverages such as milk, water, and juice. When in doubt, do without!

If you are a caffeine junkie, cutting back or cutting out caffeine can be difficult and may cause headaches and fatigue. Cut back gradually.

At the Doctor's or Midwife's Office

There will be more of the same this month as your provider checks your weight and fundal height, listens to your baby's heartbeat, and finds out about any new pregnancy symptoms you may be experiencing. Your doctor or midwife will also require the usual urine sample and blood pressure check.

If you weren't given an oral glucose tolerance test to screen for gestational diabetes last month, it will probably be administered now.

PRENATAL VISIT NOTES

Stats

Weight
....

Week of pregnancy
....

Fundal height
....

Blood pressure
....

Baby's heart rate
....

Tests

Test	Result
....	....
....	....
....	....
....	....

Additional Notes

....

....

....

....

Birth Plan Checklist

Now is a good time to go through a birth plan checklist. A birth plan is a road map for your entire childbirth experience, beginning to end. It's your chance to let everyone involved (doctors, nurses, partners) know what you want the experience to be. Use your birth plan to chart the course of labor and delivery, but remember you may have to take alternate routes occasionally depending on conditions.

1. Where will the birth take place?
   — Hospital
   — Birthing center
   — Home
   — Other:

2. Who will be there for labor support?
   — Husband or significant other
   — Doula
   — Friend
   — Family member

3. Will any room modifications or equipment be required to increase your mental and physical comfort?
   — Objects from home, such as pictures and a blanket and pillow
   — Lighting adjustments
   — Music
   — Video or photos of birth
   — Other:

4. Do you have any special requests for labor prep procedures?
   — Forgo enema
   — Forgo shaving
   — Shave self
   — Heparin lock instead of routine IV line
   — Other:

5. What do you want to eat and drink during labor?
   — A light snack
   — Water, sports drink, or other appropriate beverage
   — Ice chips
   — Other:

6. Do you want pain medication?
   — Analgesic, such as Stadol, Demerol, or Nubain
   — Epidural
   — Other:

7. What nonpharmaceutical pain relief equipment might you want access to?
   — Hydrotherapy, such as a shower or whirlpool
   — Warm compresses
   — Birth ball
   — Other:

8. What interventions would you like to avoid unless deemed a medical necessity by your provider during labor? Specify your preferred alternatives.
   — Episiotomy
   — Forceps
   — Internal fetal monitoring
   — Pitocin (oxytocin)
   — Other:

9. What would you like your first face to face with your baby to be like?
   — Hold off on all nonessential treatment, evaluation, and tests for a specified time.
   — If immediate tests and evaluation are necessary, you, your partner, or another support person will accompany the baby.
   — Want to nurse immediately following birth.
   — Would like family members to meet the baby immediately following birth.
   — Other:

10. If a Caesarean section is required, what is important to you and your partner?
   — Type of anesthesia (e.g., general vs. spinal block)
   — Having partner or another support person present
   — Spending time with the baby immediately following procedure
   — Bonding with the baby in the recovery room
   — Type of postoperative pain relief and nursing considerations
   — Other:

11. Do you have a preference for who cuts the cord?
   — You
   — Your partner
   — Provider

12. When would you like the cut to be performed?
   — Delay until cord stops pulsing.
   — Cord blood will be banked. Cut and stored per banking guidelines.
   — Cut at provider's discretion.
   — Other:

13. What kind of postpartum care will you and the baby have at the hospital?
   — Baby will room-in with mom.
   — Baby will sleep in the nursery at night.
   — Baby will breastfeed.
   — Baby will bottle feed.
   — Baby will not be fed any supplemental formula and/or glucose water unless medically indicated.
   — Baby will not be given a pacifier.
   — Other:

14. What are your considerations for after discharge?
   — Support and short-term care for siblings
   — Support if you've had a Caesarean
   — Maternity leave
   — Other:

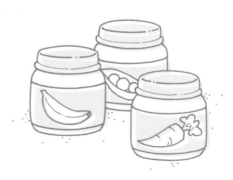

Thinking of Names

You and your significant other have no doubt been thinking about the potential name you will choose depending on the gender of the baby. To get you started on ideas, below are the most popular names for babies born in 2010.

Boys' Names	Girls' Names
Jacob	Isabella
Ethan	Sophia
Michael	Emma
Jayden	Olivia
William	Ava
Alexander	Emily
Noah	Abigail
Daniel	Madison
Aiden	Chloe
Anthony	Mia

Source: U.S. Social Security Administration

BABY NAMES—BOYS

Here you can record boys' names that you and your partner like.

....

....

....

....

....

....

....

....

....

....

....

....

....

....

....

....

....

BABY NAMES—GIRLS

Here you can record girls' names that you and your partner like.

....

....

....

....

....

....

....

....

....

....

....

....

....

....

....

....

....

MILESTONES

Here is a place for you to record the thoughts, feelings, and physical changes you experience during your sixth month of pregnancy.

Time until due date: _____

Firsts:

....

....

....

Concerns:

....

....

....

Looking forward to:

....

....

....

Questions for the doctor or midwife next month:

....

....

....

Journal

Date :   /   /

Dear Daughter (or Son): Write your future 16-year-old child a letter. What are your hopes and dreams for them? How are you feeling as you progress through your pregnancy?

Journal

Date :   /   /

Journal

Date :   /   /

Journal

Date :   /   /

PART 8

Month Seven

You're likely feeling perpetually stuffed and slightly out of breath as your uterus relocates all your internal organs. The relief and energy felt in the second trimester may start to fade now. Just remember, you're almost there!

Month Seven Checklist

✓ Make a date with yourself to relax, read, or just catch up on sleep.
✓ Interview pediatricians.
✓ Sign up for childbirth classes.
✓ Contemplate the breast versus bottle decision.
✓ Set up an appointment to discuss your birth plan with your provider.

Your Baby This Month

Weighing in at 4 pounds and about 16" long, your baby is growing amazingly fast now. His red, wrinkled skin is losing its fine lanugo covering as more insulating fat accumulates. And his eyelids, closed for so long, can now open and afford him a dim view of the place he will call home for just a few more months.

Dramatic developments in the brain and central nervous system are also occurring. Your baby feels pain, can cry, and responds to stimulation from light or sound outside the womb. Periodically, tiny elbows and feet will turn your belly into an interactive relief map.

Your Body's Changes

The top of the fundus is halfway between your belly button and your breastbone, displacing your stomach, intestines, and diaphragm.

Your breasts are heavier and more glandular and are getting ready to feed your baby. In this last trimester, your nipples may begin to leak colostrum, which is the yellowish, nutrient-rich fluid that precedes real breast milk. To reduce backaches and breast tenderness, make sure you wear a well-fitting bra (even to bed if it helps). If you are planning on breastfeeding, you may want to start buying the following few things now that can take you through the rest of pregnancy.

- **Nursing bra:** Try out the clasps for easy nursing access. Try to unfasten and slip the nursing flaps down with one hand.
- **Sports bra:** Instead of a nursing bra, you may opt for the comfort of a sports bra that slides up easily.
- **Easy-access shirts:** Button-up blouses, shirts with zippers, and other easy-access clothing will make nursing easier on a day-to-day basis.
- **Nursing pads:** These pads, which catch leaks before they soak through your shirt, come in several different materials and configurations, including cloth, plastic, and disposable.

If you will not be breastfeeding but using formula or bottle-feeding breast milk instead, look for a bottle with these characteristics:

- **Low air flow:** Designs that minimize air or can be de-aired prior to feeding may reduce your baby's gas.
- **Convenience:** If saving time is a priority, features like presterilized disposable bag bottles are a big plus.
- **Easy to clean:** Pick something with minimal parts that looks relatively easy to clean and sterilize.
- **Built for baby:** Make sure your baby gets a newborn-style nipple with a smaller opening to start so he doesn't face a formula tidal wave. If his sucking reflex is weak, however, you may have to upgrade to a larger opening.

Your body is warming up for labor, and you may start to experience Braxton Hicks contractions. These painless and irregular contractions feel as if your uterus is making a fist and then gradually relaxing it. If your little one is fairly active, you may think that he is stretching himself sideways at first. A quick check of your belly may reveal a visible tightening.

Braxton Hicks can begin as early as week twenty and continue right up until your due date, although they're more commonly felt in the final month of pregnancy.

The list is growing. Other symptoms that may continue this month include:

— Fatigue
— Frequent urination
— Tender and/or swollen breasts
— Bleeding gums
— Excess mucus and saliva
— Increase in vaginal discharge
— Mild shortness of breath
— Lightheadedness or dizziness
— Headaches
— Forgetfulness
— Gas
— Heartburn
— Constipation
— Skin and hair changes
— Round ligament pain or soreness
— Lower back aches
— Mild swelling of legs, feet, and hands
— Leg cramps

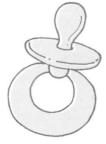

On Your Mind

You may now be wondering whether you are up to the task of labor and whether you will be up to the task of motherhood.

Remember that women have been doing this since the beginning of time, and under much more difficult circumstances. In most cases labor will be hard work, but if you prepare yourself by learning what to expect, you will be ready to face whatever comes your way.

Also keep in mind that great moms are made, not born. While some parts of mothering will seem to come to you instinctively, practice and trial and error will make up the better part of your parenting education. Use the tools around you—your pediatrician, other mothers, and research and reading—to build and sharpen your skills, but listen to your inner voice in the final analysis and application of what you learn.

Eating for Two

Getting enough calcium is especially important in the third trimester, when your baby's bones and teeth are rapidly developing. While your prenatal supplement should give you and baby most of what you need, ensure that your diet includes a healthy balance of calcium-rich foods like milk, yogurt, broccoli, greens, and calcium-fortified breakfast cereals and beverages.

If you aren't getting enough calcium in food and supplements, your baby will draw on your calcium stores in your body, which could increase your risk of developing osteoporosis later in life. Check your supplement and make sure you're getting 1,000 mg of calcium daily. However, keep in mind that too much calcium isn't a good thing either, as it can inhibit the absorption of iron. Keep your intake below 2,500 mg daily from supplement and food sources.

At the Doctor's or Midwife's Office

Starting with this initial third-trimester visit, your visits to the doctor may start to step up to twice monthly. Women who are Rh negative will need treatment with *Rh immunoglobulin (RhIg)* this month. An injection is typically given at about twenty-eight weeks to protect the fetus from developing hemolytic disease—a condition in which the mother's antibodies attack the fetal red blood cells.

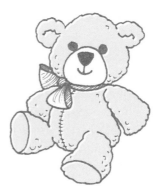

Choosing a Pediatrician

Your pediatrician will look in on and care for your newborn in the hospital, so getting one lined up now is important. Some things to inquire about beyond the basic office hours and insurance questions include:

Do ill children have a waiting room separate from the one for well-child visits?

....

....

Will the doctor support your feeding choice?

....

....

Are lactation consultants available?

....

....

How are calls into the office triaged and returned?

....

....

Additional questions or concerns:

....

....

Arranging Child Care

Now is also a good time to begin scoping out potential child care providers. Your best source of leads for good child care is other moms in your life who share your values and viewpoints on child rearing. Then narrow down your list of facilities based on the answers to the following questions. You should visit and observe children at any facility you are considering for your own child.

1. Does the facility have adequate staffing? (For infants, this is generally a minimum of one provider to every three babies.)

    ....

    ....

    ....

    ....

    ....

2. Does the facility provide a stimulating and child-friendly environment?

    ....

    ....

    ....

    ....

    ....

3. What is the staff like? (Are they caring and nurturing, or do they seem to be distracted or overburdened?)

....

....

....

....

4. Is the facility properly licensed and accredited? (See the website of the National Association for the Education of Young Children, *http://www.naeyc.org*, if you are unsure.)

....

....

....

....

5. Is an adequate number of the staff specially trained for early childhood care?

....

....

....

....

6. Do the children in the program seem comfortable and happy?

....

....

....

7. Are parents allowed to observe when their child is in the program?

....

....

....

8. Does the program focus on emotional, cognitive, and physical development in activities?

....

....

....

9. Does the staff provide adequate individual attention to infants?

....

....

....

....

....

MILESTONES

Here is a place for you to record the thoughts, feelings, and physical changes you experience during your seventh month of pregnancy.

Time until due date: _____

Firsts:

....

....

....

Concerns:

....

....

....

Looking forward to:

....

....

....

Questions for the doctor or midwife next month:

....

....

....

Journal

Date :   /   /

Your Belly: How are you feeling about your changing body? Is your growing baby bump something you're enjoying, or are you still trying to get used to your burgeoning belly? Is baby moving around a lot? How did that first "kick" feel?

Journal

Date :   /   /

Journal

Date :   /   /

Journal

Date :   /   /

Journal

Date :   /   /

PART 9

Month Eight

You are a pregnancy pro now, deftly handling all the aches and pains that come with the territory. You've learned to adjust to the fashion hardships, the lifestyle changes, and the logistical challenges that your baby and belly have brought to the forefront. It's not much longer now.

Month Eight Checklist

✓ Take five and de-stress; it's good for you and baby.
✓ Lay out your baby's essentials.
✓ Compare and decide on cloth versus disposal diapers.
✓ Discuss circumcision with your pediatrician and your partner.
✓ Start wrapping up projects at work.
✓ Finalize your child care plans for after maternity leave.
✓ Preregister at your hospital or birthing center.

Your Baby This Month

Gradually shifting to the same position in which 95 percent of all babies are born, your baby starts to move into a head-down pose, known as the vertex position.

Your little one is now up to 18" long and as heavy as a 5-pound sack of flour. The rest of her body is finally catching up to the size of her head. Although it may feel like your baby is constantly up and about, she's actually sleeping 90–95 percent of the day, a figure that will drop only slightly when she is born.

If your child were born today, she'd have an excellent chance of surviving and eventually thriving outside the womb. However, she'd still be considered preterm or premature, just as any birth before thirty-seven weeks of gestation.

Your Body's Changes

Weight gain should start to slow down this month. If it doesn't, however, don't cut your calorie intake below 2,600 to try and stop it. You need the extra energy for both of you.

As your baby settles firmly on your bladder, bathroom stops step up once again. You may even experience some stress incontinence, which is minor dribbling or leakage of urine when you sneeze, cough, laugh, or make other sudden movements. This should clear up postpartum.

Other symptoms that may begin or continue this month include:

— Fatigue
— Frequent urination
— Tender and/or swollen breasts
— Colostrum discharge from nipples
— Bleeding gums
— Excess mucus and saliva
— Increase in vaginal discharge
— Mild shortness of breath
— Lightheadedness or dizziness
— Headaches
— Forgetfulness
— Gas
— Heartburn
— Constipation
— Skin and hair changes
— Round ligament pain or soreness
— Lower back aches
— Mild swelling of legs, feet, and hands
— Leg cramps

✓ Painless, irregular Braxton Hicks contractions
✓ Minor vision changes (fluid retention can slightly change the shape of your eyes and estrogen can cause your eyes to be drier than normal)

On Your Mind

As labor looms closer, your thoughts turn to the task at hand. Going into labor and delivery with as much knowledge of the process as possible can make the difference between a positive childbirth experience and a long and arduous one, so continue to read and ask questions.

Eating for Two

Restaurants can make high-calorie, big-portion temptations a little too easy to indulge in. But everyone is allowed to have the occasional night away from the kitchen—especially a mom-to-be. Smart planning can help you enjoy dining out without blowing your calorie budget.

First off, banish the bread basket. It's too easy to fill up on empty calories while you wait for your entrée. When you order, choose low-calorie salad dressings, and ask for dressing, sauces, and other condiments to be served on the side so you can control portions. Avoid fried and breaded entrées and look for options that are broiled, baked, grilled, steamed, or roasted.

Restaurant portions are often more than a single serving. As soon as you feel full, have the wait staff take your plate. If you know ahead of time that you're getting a heaping helping, consider splitting an entrée with your dining companion, or ask for a container to wrap half the entrée for a doggie bag before you start eating.

Many restaurants have their menu offerings listed online, so do a little homework before planning your night out to ensure that the place you choose has healthy options for you.

At the Doctor's or Midwife's Office

You'll see your provider twice this month as you continue your every-other-week routine. He or she will check the position of your baby to determine if she has turned head down in preparation for birth.

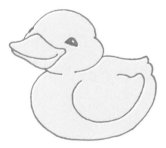

PRENATAL VISIT NOTES

Stats

Weight
....

Week of pregnancy
....

Fundal height
....

Blood pressure
....

Baby's heart rate
....

Tests

Test   Result

....

....

....

....

Additional Notes

....

....

....

....

Nesting

At this time you will probably be feeling the urge to make your home as cozy and welcoming for your baby as possible. Here are some baby essentials you should have on the shelves prior to her arrival:

— Diapers
— Wipes
— Alcohol swabs (for her umbilical cord)
— Baby shampoo
— Baby soap
— Diaper rash ointment
— Waterproof pads (for cutting down on laundry)
— Bottles (even if you're breastfeeding you may pump milk occasionally)
— Thermometer
— Infant Tylenol or another fever-reducing product as recommended by your pediatrician
— Baby blankets

The Diaper Debate

Deciding whether you'd like to use cloth diapers or disposable diapers is a choice many new mothers go back and forth on. Some moms swear by the old-fashioned and eco-friendly use of cloth diapers, while others find the convenience of disposable diapers a necessity. Your decision may depend on a variety of factors, including your concern about the environment, the amount of time and labor you are willing to devote to maintaining a supply of clean diapers, and the level of convenience that would work best for you from day to day.

Below you will find a list of pros and cons to help you decide where you stand in the cloth versus disposable diaper debate.

Using Cloth Diapers

Pros
Biodegradable
Cheaper than plastic
Can be less irritating for baby's skin

Cons
Requires electricity and water to wash
Can become expensive if you hire a service to wash diapers
Labor intensive if you wash them yourself

Call local diaper services to get estimates and a run-down of what's included.

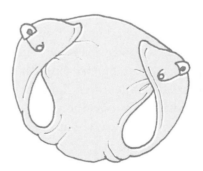

CLOTH DIAPER SERVICE RESEARCH

Service name

Phone number

Address

Cost per week

Services included for cost

Service name

Phone number

Address

Cost per week

Services included for cost

Service name

Phone number

Address

Cost per week

Services included for cost

Service name

Phone number

Address

Cost per week

Services included for cost

Service name

Phone number

Address

Cost per week

Services included for cost

Service name

Phone number

Address

Cost per week

Services included for cost

Planning for the postpartum period can be a tremendous help in getting organized after you and your baby are back at home.

Will you have live-in help (other than that from your partner) for a few days or weeks?

....

Helper Contact Info

Helper's name:
....

Helper's phone number:
....

Helper's e-mail address:
....

Helper's address:
....

....

Dates and times available to help:

....

....

....

Have you arranged childcare for the baby's siblings?

....

....

....

Caretaker Contact Info

Caretaker's name:
....

Caretaker's phone number:
....

Caretaker's e-mail address:
....

Caretaker's address:
....

Dates and times available to watch siblings:

....

....

Scheduled Time Off

Are you and your partner both taking time off?

....

Dates of your time off:

....

....

....

Dates of your partner's time off:

....

....

....

Here is a place for you to record the thoughts, feelings, and physical changes you experience during your eighth month of pregnancy.

Time until due date: _____

Firsts:

....

....

....

Concerns:

....

....

....

Looking forward to:

....

....

....

Questions for the doctor or midwife next month:

....

....

....

Journal

Date :   /   /

Nesting: Have you finished preparing your baby's new space? Is there a special theme for the nursery? What other ways have you started preparing your home for the arrival of the newest member of your family?

Journal

Date :   /   /

Journal

Date :   /   /

Journal

Date :   /   /

Journal

Date :   /   /

Journal

Date :   /   /

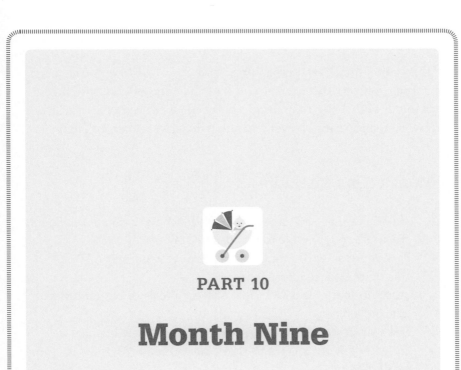

PART 10

Month Nine

The grand finale is approaching. You may feel like you've been waiting forever. But even if you had the time of conception pinpointed, your baby may decide he needs a little more, or a little less, time preparing. Never fear; he will arrive sooner or later.

Month Nine Checklist

✓ Make sure that your other children's teachers and care providers are aware of your impending hospital stay.
✓ Pack your bag and compile a call list for your partner.
✓ Line up postpartum assistance.
✓ Stock up the freezer with heat-and-eat meals or recruit postpartum kitchen help.
✓ Make a plan, and a backup plan, for getting to the hospital.
✓ Put your feet up, relax, and take a deep breath. The rest is up to your baby!

Your Baby This Month

Your child is packing on about ½ pound per week as he prepares to make his big exit. He's fully formed and just waiting for the right time now. His lungs, the last organ system to fully mature, now have an adequate level of surfactant in them to allow for breathing outside of the womb.

Your Body's Changes

While your baby is still growing, your weight gain tapers off, and you may even lose a pound or so due to a drop in amniotic fluid production. Many more things are happening this month. Check off those you experience, note when they occur, and call your doctor or midwife with any questions.

— Groin soreness
— Backache
— As your cervix thins and dilates (opens), the soft mucous plug keeping it sealed tight may be dislodged
— Increased need to urinate
— Feel shockwaves through your pelvis as your baby settles further down onto the pelvic floor

Braxton Hicks contractions may be more frequent this month as you draw nearer to delivery. You're close enough to be on the lookout for the real thing, however. You know you are experiencing real contractions when they:

• Are felt in the back and possibly radiate around to the abdomen.
• Do not subside when you move around or change positions.
• Increase in intensity with activity like walking.
• Increase in intensity as time passes.
• Come at roughly regular intervals (early on this may be from twenty to forty-five minutes apart).

Other signs that labor is on its way include amniotic fluid leaks in either a gush or a trickle (your water breaking), sudden diarrhea, and the appearance of the mucous plug. For many women, the bag of waters does not break until active labor sets in.

On Your Mind

You're likely tired but happy as you pack and prepare for the big day. Just remember the "estimated" in estimated delivery date to avoid a big letdown if baby is tardy.

As sleep gets more and more elusive and your discomfort increases, you may find yourself easily provoked. To keep your cool and limit anxiety:

- Stay clear of encounters with people you know will irritate you.
- Ask your significant other to be the point person on all "anything yet?" questions.
- Take a deep breath and go over what you learned in childbirth class.
- Talk with your partner or labor coach about ways to relax.
- Ask your provider any questions that may still be on your mind about labor and delivery.

Eating for Two

For years, doctors would only allow ice chips to pass the lips of moms in labor. But labor is hard, energy-consuming work, and contemporary medicine has recognized that the ice-chip mandate is too restrictive for most women at low risk of labor complications. Most physicians and midwives now allow women to at least consume fluids liberally throughout labor, and some may even give consideration to approved snacks. If you haven't discussed this issue with your healthcare provider yet, it's a good idea to get their guidelines (or the hospital guidelines) at your next prenatal appointment.

Clear liquids are considered acceptable throughout labor by most doctors and midwives. Water is always a good idea to stay hydrated, and the added carbohydrates in sports drinks and fruit juices make them good options as well. While there's no medical reason not to drink seltzer or soft drinks in labor, you might opt out of fizzy drinks to avoid gas. If you feel famished but your doctor says solid food is a no-no, fluids like clear broths and ice pops may help take the edge off your hunger.

You can and should nourish yourself in early labor, before checking in at the hospital or birthing center. Although you may not feel like eating, it's critical to keep your energy stores up for the marathon ahead. Follow these general guidelines for snacking:

- **Forgo the fat.** Steer clear of fatty foods that are slowly digested, such as meat and dairy. The same goes for gassy foods like beans and broccoli.
- **Carb load.** Carbs will help fuel your body for the task ahead. A cup of plain pasta, some crackers, or a piece of whole-grain toast with jam are all good power-packed snack ideas.
- **Graze, don't gorge.** Keep portions small and frequent versus one big meal that will tax your digestive system.

If your healthcare provider does allow snacks in later labor, opt for simple carbohydrates that are easily digested and can give you the energy bursts you need to make it to the finish line. Fruit or fruit leather, honey sticks, Jell-O, and applesauce are all tummy-friendly options.

At the Doctor's or Midwife's Office

You'll see your doctor or midwife on a weekly basis now until you deliver. You should expect that your provider will:

- Perform an internal exam with each visit to check your cervix for changes that indicate approaching labor.
- Administer a group B strep (GBS) test one month prior to your estimated delivery date.
- Take note of any descent or dropping of the baby toward the pelvis. This descent is called the pelvic station.

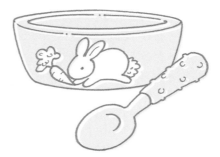

PRENATAL VISIT NOTES

Stats

Weight
....

Week of pregnancy
....

Fundal height
....

Blood pressure
....

Baby's heart rate
....

Tests

Test	Result
....	....
....	....
....	....
....	....

Additional Notes

....

....

....

....

Gearing Up for the Big Event

Since a baby's timetable is somewhat unpredictable, start getting your affairs in order at the beginning of this month. Make sure to:

— Double-check with your doctor or midwife that a copy of your birth plan has been put into your chart.

— See that your birth plan includes any changes you might have made to it since your first review together.

— Provide your labor coach with an extra copy of your birth plan just in case the original is misplaced.

— Take up friends, family, and neighbors on their offers of assistance. Make a list and schedule assignments (see the chart that follows to compile this list).

— Give friends who are good in the kitchen cooking detail, so you can have a supply of frozen, home-cooked meals on hand for easy dinners.

— If you have other children, charge your husband or partner with making sure their school, extracurricular, and social schedules are covered.

— Sound out the idea with your partner of asking a mommy expert, maybe even your own mom, to come for a visit.

When family and friends offer to help you after the baby is born, first make sure they are making genuine offers. If they really do intend to help, take them up on their kindness! Allow these goodhearted people to take pets for walks, pick up groceries, or, if you have other children, to help you look after them. To keep track of the offers of family and friends to help you and your partner out postpartum, use this space to record the details.

Task	Individual Volunteering	Times Available to Help
....	....	....
....	....	....
....	....	....
....	....	....
....	....	....
....	....	....
....	....	....
....	....	....
....	....	....
....	....	....

Packing Your Bag

Essentials you should pack for your delivery include:

Pain-relief tools for labor: Include things like massage balls, a picture for focusing on through contractions, a water bottle, and so forth.

Music to labor by: Check with your hospital or birthing center in advance to see if a small portable stereo is acceptable. If not, you can always bring personal headphones.

Snacks: If your hospital or birthing center allows food and/or drink in labor, pack yourself a small cooler with supplies. And don't forget about a little something for your coach.

Stopwatch, clock, or watch with a second hand: This will come in handy for timing contractions.

Camera: For capturing baby's arrival (or the moments shortly thereafter), don't forget the batteries and film (or an extra memory card)!

Phone numbers: Make sure your partner has names and numbers of the folks you'll want to clue in immediately on the new arrival.

Several nightgowns: Bring some with button or snap fronts if you're going to nurse.

Extra underwear: Make them comfortable but not your best. They'll probably end up with some postpartum bloodstains.

Sanitary pads: The hospital will provide you with some, but extras are good to have on hand.

Picture of the kids: If you have other children, taping a picture of big brother or sister to your newborn's bassinet is a good way to emphasize your first child's important new role in the family.

Glasses or contacts: Make sure you can see the baby after he's finally here.

Warm socks and/or slippers: Those hospital floors can be cold.

Bathrobe: You'll want this for hallway walks to the nursery.

Toiletries: Remember toothbrush, toothpaste, and other basics.

Shower supplies: You'll be given an opportunity to shower at the hospital, so pack shampoo and other necessities.

Going-home outfits for both you and your baby: Pack a set of newborn clothes and make sure you bring something loose and comfortable to wear yourself.

Baby blanket: You'll want to swaddle your baby for his return home. Let your partner bring the car seat on discharge day so you aren't overwhelmed with luggage.

If you're breastfeeding, you might also pack:

Nursing bras: If you don't have any yet, a bra with a front fastener will work well as a stand-in for now.

Box of nursing pads: These will be handy for when your milk comes in.

Vitamin E oil or lanolin ointment: Pack them for sore or cracked nipples.

Additional Items to Bring:

....

....

....

....

Outfitting Your Baby

In addition to some of the other products you may have purchased in anticipation of baby's arrival (diapers, wipes, car seat, alcohol swabs, baby shampoo, baby soap, bottles, and a thermometer), make sure you have the following before you bring your new baby home:

— Three undershirts that snap
— Ten onesies and/or one-piece sleepers (depending on the season and climate you live in)
— Five bibs with waterproof linings (e.g., rubber)
— Three hooded bath towels
— Seven pairs of booties or socks
— Ten+ towels or cloth diapers for dealing with spitup
— Four+ snap-up jumpsuits for daywear
— Two+ baby hats
— Nightlight
— Baby monitor
— Four+ crib or bassinet sheets
— Four+ receiving blankets
— Baby nail clippers
— Four+ face cloths
— Q-tips and/or cotton balls
— Baby oil
— Diaper rash ointment
— Changing pad

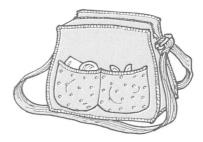

Items for Leaving the House

Once you and your baby are home from the hospital, you'll need a few items so that you can pay visits to friends and family (and be out and about) with everything you'll need to keep you and your baby comfortable. Some items you might consider purchasing are:

- Stroller
- Jogging stroller
- Diaper bag
- Backpack or convertible backpack/frontpack
- Car seat
- Toy for car seat
- Sling
- Sunshade

Additional Items to Buy:

....

....

....

....

....

....

....

....

....

Here you can record the contact information for those people your partner or labor coach should call immediately when your baby is born to share the good news.

Person's Name	Phone Number	E-mail Address	Successfully Contacted?
....	....	....	....
....	....	....	....
....	....	....	....
....	....	....	....
....	....	....	....
....	....	....	....
....	....	....	....
....	....	....	....
....	....	....	....
....	....	....	....
....	....	....	....
....	....	....	....
....	....	....	....

Record the contact information for anyone you want to send a birth announcement to.

Name:
....

Phone number:
....

E-mail address:
....

Address:
....

....

Name:
....

Phone number:
....

E-mail address:
....

Address:
....

....

....

Name:
....

Phone number:
....

E-mail address:
....

Address:
....

....

....

Name:
....

Phone number:
....

E-mail address:
....

Address:
....

....

....

Name:
....

Phone number:
....

E-mail address:
....

Address:
....

....

....

Name:
....

Phone number:
....

E-mail address:
....

Address:
....

....

....

Name:

....

Phone number:

....

E-mail address:

....

Address:

....

....

....

Name:

....

Phone number:

....

E-mail address:

....

Address:

....

....

....

Name:

....

Phone number:

....

E-mail address:

....

Address:

....

....

....

LABOR-TIME CHECKLIST FOR YOUR PARTNER

Remembering everything in the thrill of the big moment may be hard, so make a checklist and keep it on your car's dashboard so that you remember everything when the time comes. Also remember to top off your gas tank every time it gets below the halfway mark, so that you won't have to make a stop for gas on the way to the hospital.

○ Overnight bag

○ Cell phone, calling card, or plenty of quarters for pay-phone calls (if cell phones are not allowed to be used in the hospital)

○ Phone number list

○ ....

○ ....

○ ....

○ ....

○ ....

○ ....

○ ....

○ ....

○ ....

○ ....

○ ....

○ ....

○ ....

BABY GIFTS

Be sure to record the sender and gift item for all baby gifts you receive. That way you will have an easy reference for when you are well rested and ready to send out thank-you cards!

Gift Item	Sender	Date Card Mailed

BABY GIFTS (continued)

Gift Item	Sender	Date Card Mailed

LABOR AND DELIVERY

Time of first contraction:
....

Where you were when labor began:
....

Date admitted:
....

Time admitted:
....

Delivery date:
....

Delivery time:
....

Baby's length:
....

Baby's weight:
....

Any complications during labor and delivery:
....

....

....

Additional information about delivery:
....

....

....

....

....

....

....

....

Here is a place for you to record the thoughts, feelings, and physical changes you experience during your ninth month of pregnancy.

Time until due date: _____

Firsts:

....

....

....

Concerns:

....

....

....

Looking forward to:

....

....

....

Questions for the doctor or midwife next month:

....

....

....

Journal

Date :   /   /

The Big Event: How are you feeling about your impending labor and delivery? Nervous? Excited? A little of both? What is your biggest fear of, and your greatest hope for, the experience?

Journal

Date :   /   /

Journal

Date :   /   /

Journal

Date :   /   /

PART 11

Bringing Baby Home

The first days at home with your new family are fun but challenging. Your body is going through some intense physical changes. Enjoy this special time getting acquainted and settling into your new lifestyle.

Your Body Postpartum

From the moment your child slides out of your body, a transformation as dramatic as that of pregnancy begins. Right at delivery you will drop around 10–15 pounds of baby, placenta, amniotic fluid, and lochia.

By the tenth day postpartum, your uterus will have contracted to one-twentieth of its prelabor size and the cervix will be closed once again. Afterpains similar to menstrual cramps and a steady discharge of lochia indicate that the uterus is returning to normal. The lochia flow will continue up to six weeks, but the afterpains will probably stop several days after delivery (although nursing may continue to stimulate them periodically). Your perineal area may continue to be sore for a few weeks. Some things you can use to ease pain and swelling are:

- A hot water bottle
- The peribottle you may have received at the hospital
- Occasional cold packs
- A foam "donut" from a medical supply store for your chair (if sitting is uncomfortable)

As your body drops tissue and fluids and decreases its cardiovascular volume, your metabolism may seem out of whack. In addition, you may find the following:

- Vaginally, things may seem a little "looser." Vaginal skin is elastic, and may be stretched out from the birth. Exercise and time will help it return to a firmer state.
- Constipation is another common postpartum problem. Plenty of water, movement, and high-fiber foods may help.
- Your breasts will be tender as you deal with engorgement. If you breastfeed, sore nipples and other discomforts may be plaguing you as you adjust to this new routine.

Recovering after Caesarean

When you've had a C-section you're recovering from major surgery and need to treat yourself accordingly.

- Sleep when baby sleeps and stay away from strenuous activity and heavy lifting (nothing bigger than baby as a general rule).
- Use a bed pillow or a nursing pillow to hold your baby without pressuring your incision.
- Pain medication may be prescribed; if you're breastfeeding, talk to your doctor about judicious use.
- Your doctor will recommend six weeks of rest and recuperation and you'll be advised not to drive while taking pain medications.
- Above all, don't push it, or you'll set your recovery back even further.

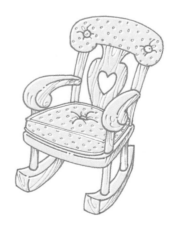

Your Baby's Body

Your baby will actually lose weight as she starts out in life, but should be back up to birth weight by her two-week checkup. Thereafter, she may put on 1 pound every two weeks, doubling her birth weight by month four. Premature babies sometimes grow a little slower, but most will eventually catch up.

Reflexes

Your newborn arrives with a variety of natural reflexes or involuntary ways of moving:

- **Palmar, or grasping, reflex.** When you touch your baby's open hand, she'll make a fist around your finger.
- **Rooting reflex.** If you stroke her cheek, her head will turn toward your touch. This reflex helps your newborn find her food source.
- **Sucking reflex.** Once at the breast or bottle, your baby's sucking reflex takes over as she automatically sucks on anything put in her mouth.
- **Startle, or moro, reflex.** When your baby is startled, he will thrust his arms and legs out and arch his back, then quickly pull arms and legs in again.
- **Babinski reflex.** Stroking your baby's foot will make him spread his toes and flex his foot in.
- **Stepping reflex.** If you hold your baby up with your hands under her armpits so that her feet are touching a firm surface, she will lift her feet up and down.
- **Tonic neck reflex.** When placed on his back, baby turns his head to the right and makes fists with his hands.
- **Blinking.** The involuntary reflex of closing her eyes when they are exposed to bright light, air, or another stimulus is the one reflex that your baby will keep for the rest of her life.

Birthmarks

Your baby may be born with one or more birthmarks:

- **Salmon patches or "stork bites."** Red marks on the eyelids, forehead, and at the very back of the nape of the neck usually fade and disappear over time.
- **Hemangioma or strawberry birthmarks.** These red, slightly raised marks can increase in size but may shrink and be gone by age five.
- **Café au lait spots.** Light brown birthmarks. Very rarely, large numbers of these birthmarks are symptomatic of medical conditions. Talk to your child's doctor if you have any concerns.
- **Mongolian spots.** Dark blue to blue-green spots on the buttocks or lower back are most common in African American, Native American, and Asian newborns, and many fade over time.
- **Port wine stains.** Bright red or purple marks that are considered to be more permanent. Laser removal is an option in later life if they are located in a prominent spot.
- **Milia.** Little whiteheads called milia are common on newborns, especially around the nose, and may come and go during the first few days.
- **Petechia.** These are red to purple pinpoints that you may see on your baby's face from the trauma of coming down the birth canal. These will disappear in a few days.

The Umbilical Cord

Baby's umbilical cord stump looks like a dark, dried up protrusion. You'll be instructed to:

- Clean it regularly, usually with alcohol swabs
- Keep it dry to prevent breakage and bleeding
- Keep an eye open for signs of infection, such as pus or inflammation

Within two weeks or so, the stump will fall off and your baby's perfect little belly button will be revealed.

Breast or Bottle?

Are you going to breastfeed or go the formula route? If you were comparing breast milk to formula strictly on a nutrient basis, few would disagree that the best choice is breast milk. But since the issue is also loaded with social, emotional, and personal considerations, things are seldom so black and white. In the end, breast or bottle is an individual choice.

Your Body and Breastfeeding

With all nursing positions, make sure your baby's head is well supported. After you're settled into position, brace your breast with one hand, cupped into the shape of a "C." Encouraging baby to get a successful latch is the most important part of the process. Stroke her bottom lip with your nipple until she opens her mouth wide and yawn-like. This is called the rooting reflex. Insert your nipple into her mouth and she should instinctively close, or latch, onto it. A proper latch:

- Encompasses the entire nipple and most, if not all, of the areola
- Positions her nose almost directly on your breast
- Can be verified by her visible and possibly audible swallowing
- Will not hurt (unless the nipple is in poor condition to begin with)

In the first few days following birth, your breasts will produce a clear to yellow sticky substance called colostrum. Colostrum contains antibodies that help strengthen the infant immune system. It also is important for getting baby's digestion off on the right track. The low-carbohydrate, high-protein concoction is easily digestible for these early days and helps to establish beneficial bacteria in your baby's gastrointestinal tract.

Colostrum comes out in small amounts compared to later breast milk. You'll know when your milk "comes in" because your breasts will become:

- Engorged with milk
- Very hard
- Sore to the touch

Nursing your baby will relieve some of the pressure quickly, although it's possible you may need a little additional help to ease soreness.

Simple but effective pain relief options include:

- Cold compresses between feedings
- Warm compresses
- Gentle breast massage
- Refrigerated cabbage leaves, draped over the breast, inside bra
- Warm showers

Breastfeeding Pros and Cons

PRO: Breast milk is custom-made for your child's nutritional needs and provides essential antibodies.
CON: If you have a medical condition that requires drug treatment, it's possible your medication may pass into breast milk.

PRO: Breastfeeding is a low-maintenance feeding routine. Never needs mixing, warming, or other preparation.
CON: You will always need to be close at hand. Breastfeeding can be physically taxing.

PRO: Nursing gives you special one-on-one bonding time with baby.
CON: No one else can pitch in on the feeding duties.

PRO: Breastfeeding is a big cost cutter. Aside from the high cost of formula, you can save on bottles, bags, and other formula-feeding purchases.
CON: You may have to purchase or rent a breast pump and buy a personal kit to use with it, which can be costly.

PRO: Many women who breastfeed experience faster postpartum weight loss.
CON: Although you may be taking your figure back, your breasts belong to baby—leaks, sore nipples, and all.

Bottle Feeding Pros and Cons

PRO: Feeding isn't only mom, all day and all night.
CON: The special mother-child bond and skin-to-skin contact that breastfeeding brings may be harder to achieve.

PRO: You can give your baby a bottle just about anywhere, anytime without feeling self-conscious or raising eyebrows.
CON: Make sure you pack sterilized bottles and nipples, formula, bottled water for mixing, a can opener for opening formula concentrate, and more.

PRO: No worries about keeping up your milk supply when you return to work.
CON: You may miss out on a golden opportunity to spend special nursing time together at home once your work schedule starts.

PRO: You can assume control of your body again.

CON: After so many months as one, you're suddenly severing a close physical bond that nursing can prolong.

Eating for Breastfeeding

The healthy eating habits you developed in pregnancy should continue to serve you and baby well during breastfeeding. Stay on track with a well-balanced diet with plenty of whole grains, fresh fruits and vegetables, and lean protein foods.

Vitamins B_6 and B_{12} requirements go up slightly during breastfeeding, but other vitamin and mineral needs stay similar to prepregnancy levels. Your provider may recommend you continue taking your prenatal supplement, or another multivitamin, while you are breastfeeding to ensure you and your baby have enough nutrients.

Calories and Weight Loss

Moms who breastfeed should eat about 500 extra calories a day over prepregnancy levels to meet your body's energy needs for breast milk production. This is particularly important in the early postpartum weeks when you are first establishing your milk supply. You can dial back your calorie intake modestly (100–200 calories) once you and baby settle into a regular breastfeeding routine to encourage postpartum weight loss.

Breastfeeding and Beverages

Keep your fluid intake up at around eight to twelve glasses of water a day. When you breastfeed, your body releases a hormone called oxytocin that can actually make many women thirsty, so it's a good idea to have a water bottle always on hand. One or two caffeine drinks a day are acceptable, but caffeine does pass into breast milk, and excessive intake can cause baby to become irritable and have difficulty sleeping.

You may choose to resume drinking alcohol now that pregnancy is over. Breastfeeding moms just need to take a few precautions to ensure their milk stays safe. Feed your baby before a planned night out or celebration, keep alcohol consumption moderate, and wait two to three hours for each drink you consume before breastfeeding baby after you drink. If you become engorged and it's been fewer than eight hours since imbibing, pump and dump your milk.

Postpartum Depression

Feeling down is a common postpartum emotion that typically passes in a few weeks. For many women, however, these feelings go beyond the basic baby blues and signal a more serious depressive or endocrine disorder.

The Baby Blues

The majority of new mothers experience what has become known as "the baby blues," a short-lived period of mild depression that appears in up to 85 percent of postpartum women. A severe shortage of sleep, disappointment with the birth experience, fluctuating hormone levels, anxieties about your baby's health and well-being, and shaky confidence in your own parenting skills can all lead to feelings of sadness and inadequacy. Fortunately, most cases of the blues resolve themselves within a few days to two weeks after birth as balance returns to the new mother's life.

More Than the Blues

Postpartum depression (PPD) occurs in about 10–15 percent of new mothers, and can drag on for up to a year. Check off any of the following symptoms if you are experiencing them and talk to your doctor about PPD:

— Feelings of extreme sadness and inexplicable crying jags
— Lack of pleasure in things you would normally enjoy
— Trouble concentrating
— Excessive worrying about the baby, or conversely, a lack of interest in the baby
— Feelings of low self-esteem
— Decreased appetite
— Feelings of resentment
— Feelings of isolation

Fortunately, PPD can be effectively treated with counseling and/or antidepressant drugs, so ask your doctor for a referral to a mental health professional.

Thyroid Problems

Thyroid problems are fairly common after childbirth, but the symptoms can be confused with other postpartum conditions. Note whether you experience any of the following common signs of postpartum thyroid conditions and contact your doctor.

— Milk supply difficulties
— Extreme fatigue
— Hair loss
— Depression

— Mood changes
— Problems losing weight
— Unusually rapid weight loss
— Heart palpitations
— Menstrual irregularities
— Sleep disorders

Some women have temporary postpartum hyperthyroidism—an overactive thyroid, with weight loss, diarrhea, racing heart, anxiety, and other symptoms of a revved-up metabolism. Doctors may prescribe drugs to ease symptoms, but this condition often resolves itself quickly. Other women can develop temporary postpartum hypothyroidism—an underactive thyroid—with fatigue, weight gain, constipation, depression, and other symptoms of a slowed-down metabolism. Again, medication may be prescribed, depending on the severity of symptoms, and frequently the thyroid will return to normal within six months to a year after the birth.

Don't Forget to Have Fun

Once you get past the fatigue, the uncertainties, and the occasional frustrations, being a new mom can be incredibly entertaining. You have a legitimate excuse to play, explore, rhyme, sing, and revisit your childhood in general. You have an adoring little person who hangs on your every word and movement and loves you unconditionally. And you get to witness all her incredible firsts as your baby learns to smile, roll over, crawl, and eventually walk and talk. In a year, this postpartum time will be a distant memory. Treasure it while it's here.

POSTPARTUM DOCTOR'S VISIT

Here you can record any questions you may have for your doctor about the postpartum period, or any concerns you may wish to discuss with your provider.

Journal

Date :   /   /

Your Birth Story: How did labor begin? How did those early hours progress? When did you head to the hospital or birthing center? Was labor and delivery what you expected? And what was it like meeting your child for the first time?

_____

_____

_____

_____

_____

_____

_____

_____

_____

_____

_____

_____

_____

_____

Journal

Date :   /   /

Journal

Date :   /   /

Journal

Date :   /   /

Journal

Date :   /   /

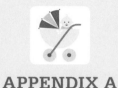

APPENDIX A

Frequently Asked Questions

Will the bottle of champagne I shared with my husband on the night we conceived our baby be harmful?
Put this night of celebration behind you and stop feeling guilty. Binge drinking or regular abuse of alcohol when you are pregnant can cause birth defects, but an isolated episode of too much champagne probably has not harmed your unborn baby.

Heavy drinking, including binges or daily use, is associated with congenital defects. Babies born with fetal alcohol syndrome (FAS) show retarded growth, have central nervous system problems, and characteristic facial features, including a small head, a thin upper lip, a short upturned nose, a flattened nasal bridge and a general underdeveloped look of the face. Because of the critical nervous system involvement, many show tremulousness, can't suck, are hyperactive, have abnormal muscle tone, and are later diagnosed with attention deficit disorder as well as mental retardation.

Relying on alcohol out of habit or cravings can also end your pregnancy abruptly. Heavy to moderate drinkers seem to experience a higher incidence of miscarriage in the second trimester, as well as problems with the placenta. Other complications linked to alcohol use are congenital heart defects, brain abnormalities, spinal and limb defects, and urinary and genital problems.

What should I take for a headache?
Most doctors say that aspirin is fine for most of your pregnancy. You should avoid it in the last month. Tylenol, or an analgesic based on acetaminophen, is also recommended for headaches, but be sure to ask your doctor before taking any medication during pregnancy.

I have terrible allergies. Is there anything my doctor is going to be able to recommend?

For some women, pregnancy can feel like a bad head cold. The increased volume of blood to your mucus membranes can make the lining of your respiratory tract swell. You may even experience nosebleeds. Fortunately, there are safe medications available to ease the symptoms, so consult with your doctor. See about taking extra vitamin C. A humidifier can also be helpful. If you experience nosebleeds as a result of allergies, try packing the nostril with gauze and then pinching your nose between your thumb and forefinger. To shrink the blood vessels and reduce bleeding, try putting an ice pack on your nose.

If I develop an infection, are there any antibiotics safe for expectant moms?

Yes. Pharmaceutical companies are coming up with new antibiotics all the time, and a number of them are safe for pregnancy. Many doctors believe that natural and synthetic penicillins are the safest antibiotics to take during pregnancy, so if you are not allergic to these oldest weapons against infection, you are definitely in luck. If you do get sick, make sure that your obstetrician is aware of anything your family doctor or another specialist may be prescribing.

What are my chances of having twins?

Your chances of "twinning" are actually not bad—about 1 in 32 births result in twins. If fraternal twins run in your family, your odds are slightly higher. The number of twins and multiple births has skyrocketed over the past several decades, with 138,660 twin births occurring in 2008. And there were 6,268 higher-order multiples—which include triplets, quadruplets, or more—born in 2008.

The Centers for Disease Control attributes approximately two-thirds of all U.S. higher-order multiples to the use of fertility treatments, also known as assisted reproductive technology (ART). Nearly 32 percent of all successful pregnancies from ART result in a multiple fraternal birth.

National statistics also reveal that more women are waiting until their thirties and forties to have children, and the increasing twin rate may reflect that reality. Women over thirty-five, especially those who have had a previous multiple birth, have an increased chance of having multiples.

You will have fraternal twins if two separate eggs are fertilized by two separate sperm. Three times more common than identical twins, and based on heredity, these fraternal fetuses have their own placentas, may even be different sexes, and may not look more like each other than ordinary brothers and sisters in the same family.

When a single fertilized egg separates into two distinct halves, identical twins are the result. These unborn babies share the same placenta, are always the same sex, and will have the same genetic makeup and similar physical characteristics.

Carrying two or more babies will put a lot more stress on your body, and your doctor is going to monitor you much more closely than if you were expecting one baby. Early detection of the babies using ultrasounds and by taking blood tests to measure your hormone levels will help keep you on track.

What are the dangers of X-rays to my unborn baby?
According to the American Academy of Family Physicians (AAFP), the maximum safe fetal radiation dose during pregnancy is 5 rad, or the equivalent of 50,000 dental X-rays or 250 mammograms. CT scans, fluoroscopic studies, and nuclear medicine tests involve slightly higher doses than conventional X-rays, but

in general still fall well within the range of acceptable exposure. In each case, the benefits of imaging need to be weighed against the potential risk to the fetus, and if at all possible, tests involving radiation should be avoided in the first trimester of pregnancy.

Can ultrasounds give misleading information?

While it's possible that you may be having a baby boy even if his external sex organs aren't visible in the ultrasound and therefore you may incorrectly think you are having a girl, most technicians won't state your baby's gender unless they are absolutely certain. If the sonogram indicates a due date that seems wrong, you might ask, "Could I possibly have dated the start of my pregnancy incorrectly?" Experts say that an ultrasound done at sixteen weeks is more accurate in regards to gestational age than an ultrasound done later in your pregnancy. When dating the length of a pregnancy, the ultrasound technician can be accurate within a few days. Ultrasounds date your pregnancy from the point of conception, which is a few days different from the point of your last period. Later ultrasounds are more accurate when determining your baby's gender. A very clear image must be obtained for the ultrasound to determine whether you are expecting a boy or a girl, and this may be more difficult to see in the early stages.

My dreams seem more vivid now that I'm pregnant. Is there a connection?

Dreams that are exceptionally realistic, disturbing, or just plain bizarre are common in pregnancy. Your dreams are reflections of what's on your mind, so it's natural for them to reflect concerns about the baby, your family, and the future. They may seem larger than life right now due to insecurities about the future, and again, those pregnancy hormones.

Why do I feel so hot and sweaty?
Your metabolism works overtime during pregnancy. Your body is burning more calories, and as a result, you often feel warm. An increase in blood supply to the surface of your skin, as well as hormones, all have an effect on how hot you feel. Keep cool by dressing in natural fibers and layering clothes so that you can always cool off by removing a layer. Hop in the shower; pat on a little talcum powder afterwards. You may need to change antiperspirants if your normal brand isn't working. To avoid dehydration as your body is working hard to burn calories and produce more blood, drink plenty of water.

Why do I often feel scatterbrained?
Increased hormones can make your thinking a bit foggy—just as they can during your menstrual cycle. Manage the situation by reducing your stress load, making lists, and going easy on yourself.

What is toxoplasmosis, and should I worry about getting it?
Toxoplasmosis is rare, but it is a virus that can affect your baby in the womb. When cats are allowed to run freely outside they can end up with a parasite that settles in the intestines and is passed on through cat feces. Toxoplasmosis can cause brain damage and other medical problems in your unborn child. Cats also frequent gardens and sandboxes, so wear gloves and wash your hands thoroughly after being outside. Don't clean any litter boxes during your pregnancy (ask your partner or a friend to help you).

Can sugar substitutes cause problems during pregnancy?
The Food and Drug Administration and the American Academy of Pediatrics agree that sucralose, aspartame, and saccharin are safe in pregnancy, but unless you have diabetes and need to control

your sugar intake, there is no good reason to consume artificial sweeteners. To be safe, limit diet drinks to one a day. However, if you are pregnant and are diagnosed with hyperphenylalanine (high levels of the amino acid phenylalanine—a component of aspartame—in your bloodstream), you should stop using the product immediately, as excessive levels of this amino acid can cause brain damage. People with the genetic disease phenylketonuria (PKU) or advanced liver disease should also avoid aspartame.

As of early 2011, sugar substitutes made with the herb stevia had not been recognized by the FDA as safe for use in pregnancy.

My doctor recommends lots of iron, but it makes me feel nauseated. What should I do?
Take iron-rich prenatal vitamin supplements between meals with plenty of water or along with a fruit juice rich in vitamin C, which enhances the absorption of iron. Avoid drinking milk, coffee, or tea with your iron supplements because these beverages inhibit iron absorption. Add liver, red meat, fish, poultry, enriched breads and cereals, green leafy vegetables, eggs, and dried fruits to your diet to increase dietary iron.

What kinds of food cravings are normal?
Many pregnant women crave sweet or salty foods. Cravings for nonfood items such as dirt, soap, ash, or coffee grounds are different. A phenomenon called pica, which has shown up in medical literature since the sixth century, results in strange cravings that can cause serious problems for a pregnant mother and her unborn baby. If you have a craving to eat clay, ashes, laundry starch, or other unusual substances, seek medical attention right away.

Can my car's seatbelt harm my unborn baby?

Definitely continue to buckle up throughout your pregnancy. The lap belt should fit snugly under your belly bulge, and the shoulder belt should be positioned between your breasts. Don't worry about your belt putting pressure on your baby. The baby is well protected by amniotic fluid and layers of tissue, muscle, and fat. It's much more dangerous to you and your child to go beltless and risk being injured in an accident.

Does intercourse hurt the baby?

Unless you have a high-risk pregnancy, you are not going to harm your baby by having sex. Sex is quite safe in a normal pregnancy. Vaginal bleeding, a history of miscarriage or premature labor, or a diagnosis of placental problems are good reasons to restrict intercourse, however. During the last month before your due date, you also should proceed with caution. Ask your practitioner if you have any concerns.

Should I circumcise my baby?

The American Academy of Pediatrics takes the stance that there is currently no firm medical or hygienic ground for performing routine circumcision (removal of the foreskin that covers the head of the penis) in newborn boys. However, the AAP also cited the importance of weighing cultural and religious beliefs and considering the child's best interest when deciding whether or not to circumcise a newborn male. If circumcision is performed, analgesia can be used to relieve the pain.

How soon can I have sex after the baby's birth?

Many doctors recommend waiting four to six weeks before having intercourse. Very few couples are able to swing back into a sex life immediately after the birth of a baby. Keep in mind either way that you can get pregnant in the period following birth. You should get back into your contraceptive routine before the mood strikes. Your doctor can give you a prescription before you leave the hospital, if necessary.

I can't stand wearing my favorite perfume anymore! Can pregnancy cause your nose to go haywire?
Pregnancy causes a heightened sensitivity to certain odors—coffee, cigarette smoke, and fried food are frequent offenders—that can contribute to stomach unrest. One theory is that these olfactory aversions are your body's way of keeping you away from substances that could harm your developing baby.

Will coloring my hair hurt my baby?
To date, there is no conclusive evidence that hair color use in pregnancy is dangerous. If you are concerned over a possible risk, you may opt for a vegetable-based or temporary color treatment until your baby is born. Some experts also recommend holding off on all chemical hair treatments during the first trimester.

I'm getting varicose veins in my legs. Is this common in pregnancy?
The hair-fine marks, also known as spider veins, usually appear on the lower legs and are caused when increased blood volume and pressure damage the valves that regulate blood flow up out of the blood vessels of the legs. The result is pooled blood in the vein and that telltale squiggly red or blue line.

Supportive stockings, putting your feet up, resting on your left side, and taking an occasional walk when you need to stand for long periods of time may relieve leg soreness associated with varicose veins.

I've had a miscarriage in the past. Is there a way to prevent it this time around?

Many miscarriages occur due to factors completely beyond anyone's control—a defective egg or sperm, or implantation outside of the endometrium. Other triggers, such as teratogen exposure, may be avoided with special precautions in pregnancy. Speak with your healthcare provider about your concerns and any special instructions given your medical history (such as restrictions on your activity).

What if I don't get to the hospital in time?

Every woman has heard stories of impatient babies being born in the backseats of taxicabs, but these impromptu deliveries are not common. Most women have plenty of time to make it to the hospital safe and sound; the average labor period runs twelve to fourteen hours. If you're concerned, you can take some basic precautions. Work out a route to the hospital in advance with your partner, keep your gas tank full, and have cash on hand for a cab just in case your car chooses the moment you go into labor to conk out.

If I'm overdue, will my provider induce me if I request it?

Whether or not to induce depends on a number of factors. Is the cervix effaced or dilated? Are you fairly sure your due date was accurate to begin with? Have you had a previous C-section? Have you had other complicating factors during pregnancy (e.g., placenta previa, umbilical cord prolapse)? Generally, if you've hit the thirty-nine-week mark, you have no history of C-section or other medical contraindications, and your provider thinks induction is indicated, she will schedule one for you.

What is umbilical cord blood banking?

Blood from the umbilical cord contains stem cells, those blank-slate cells from which all organs and tissues are built. Cord blood collected immediately after birth is placed in a collection kit and flown to a facility where it is cryogenically frozen and "banked" for later use if needed. The theory behind cord blood banking is that if your child ever develops a disease or condition requiring stem-cell treatment, the blood can be thawed and used for her treatment. If it matches certain biological markers, cord blood can be used to treat other family members as well. However, banking is cost prohibitive for many and requires an annual storage fee for as long as you would like the cord blood frozen. In recent years, some facilities have also made placenta blood banking available.

I have splotches of discolored skin on my face and abdomen. Is this normal?

Yes. Pregnancy hormones can cause hyperpigmentation of your skin, which makes certain areas of your skin (most commonly around the forehead, nose, cheeks, abdomen, and areolas) to darken. These discolored spots are usually dark on light-skinned women and light on dark-skinned women. Don't worry, though—these discolored patches will fade and eventually go away after your baby is born.

Are there exercises I should avoid during pregnancy?

Yes. A few sports are considered inappropriate during any phase of pregnancy. Mostly these sports are dangerous for reasons related to balance and risk of physical blows. It is not recommended that pregnant women ride horses, scuba dive, downhill ski, play rugby, or engage in other contact sports.

How do I know if I'm doing Kegel exercises right?
If you are doing Kegels correctly, you will not be tightening other muscles like your buttocks or thighs. You will be isolating this internal muscle and not straining other ones in the process.

Can I raise my arms above my head while pregnant?
There is an old wives' tale that says if you are pregnant, you should not lift your arms over your head. In doing so, the myth goes, you will cause your baby's umbilical cord to wrap around its neck. This is utter nonsense and should not affect how you work your arms out or move during pregnancy.

Will eating too much sugar during pregnancy lead to gestational diabetes?
No, eating too much sugar does not directly cause any type of diabetes. Diabetes is a disorder in which the body cannot properly utilize insulin or does not produce insulin, which regulates blood sugar levels. Gestational diabetes is the result of changing hormones within a woman's body.

Do folic acid supplements really make that much of a difference in preventing certain birth defects?
According to the United States Centers for Disease Control (CDC), when taken one month before conception and throughout the first trimester, folic acid supplements have been proven to reduce the risk for an NTD-affected pregnancy by 50–70 percent.

Can eating more than three times a day be part of a healthy diet?
Yes. For women who are pregnant or for anybody who enjoys a healthy lifestyle, eating several small meals during the day can fit nicely into a healthy eating pattern. It can help you to fit in those

extra calories and food group servings without having to eat large meals all at once, which can be difficult for women who may be having a problem with nausea or morning sickness.

Is it okay to take a calcium supplement if I don't eat dairy foods?
If you can't get enough calcium from the foods you choose, a supplement can be a good idea. The rule of thumb should always be food before supplements, though. First, include calcium-containing foods in your diet as much as possible, and then supplement on top of that. Never let a supplement take the place of an entire food group or nutrient such as calcium.

When should I call my doctor about a headache?
If you are in your second or third trimester and experience a bad headache, or a headache for the first time during your pregnancy, you should contact your doctor. If you have a severe headache that comes on suddenly, won't go away, and is unlike any you have ever experienced, you should call your doctor. You should contact your doctor if you have a headache that worsens and is accompanied by vision problems, speech problems, drowsiness, and/or numbness. Also call your doctor if your headache is accompanied by a stiff neck and fever.

Is it unhealthy to have an aversion to vegetables during my first trimester?
It is common for women to have food aversions even to healthy foods such as vegetables. Try drinking vegetable juice instead of eating whole vegetables. You can also eat more fruit, since many of them contain some of the same nutrients as vegetables. Keep taking your prenatal vitamins to ensure you are getting all of the nutrients that your body needs at this time. However, it's always best to get your nutrients from food before supplements. If you

have a temporary aversion to a healthy food, make substitutions. If you're not sure what to substitute, be sure to speak to a dietitian.

How can I tell whether I am experiencing morning sickness or something more serious?

If you vomit more than three or four times a day, are hardly able to keep any food down, lose weight, feel very tired and dizzy, and urinate less than usual, you may have something more serious than run-of-the-mill morning sickness—specifically, you may be suffering from hyperemesis gravidarum (HG). Additional symptoms include increased heart rate, headaches, and pale, dry-looking skin. It is important to diagnose and treat HG as soon as possible, so contact your doctor if you feel any of these symptoms or feel that your morning sickness is more serious.

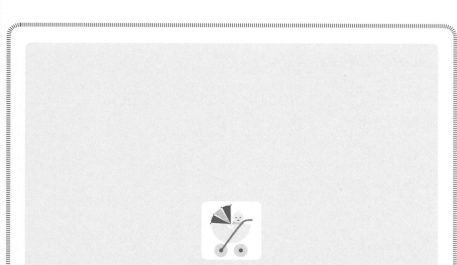

APPENDIX B

Important Contact Information

Insurance Company

Company name:
....

Policy number:
....

Phone number:
....

Address:
....

....

Office hours:
....

E-mail address:
....

Family Doctor

Name:
....

Office phone number:
....

Emergency phone number:
....

Office address:
....

....

Office hours:
....

E-mail address:
....

Gynecologist

Name:
....

Office phone number:
....

Emergency phone number:
....

Office address:
....

....

Office hours:
....

E-mail address:
....

Obstetrician

Name:
....

Office phone number:
....

Emergency phone number:
....

Office address:
....

....

Office hours:
....

E-mail address:
....

Midwife

Name:
....

Office phone number:
....

Emergency phone number:
....

Office address:
....

....

Available hours:
....

E-mail address:
....

Doula

Name:
....

Office phone number:
....

Emergency phone number:
....

Office address:
....

....

Available hours:
....

E-mail address:
....

Appendix B: Important Contact Information

Hospital

Name:
....

Phone number:
....

Emergency phone number:
....

Address:
....

....

Visiting hours:
....

E-mail address:
....

Pediatrician

Name:
....

Office phone number:
....

Emergency phone number:
....

Office address:
....

....

Office hours:
....

E-mail address:
....

Name:
....

Phone number:
....

Emergency phone number:
....

Address:
....

....

E-mail address:
....

Name:
....

Phone number:
....

Emergency phone number:
....

Address:
....

....

E-mail address:
....

Name:
....

Phone number:
....

Emergency phone number:
....

Address:
....

....

E-mail address:
....

Name:
....

Phone number:
....

Emergency phone number:
....

Address:
....

....

E-mail address:
....

Name:
....

Phone number:
....

Emergency phone number:
....

Address:
....

....

E-mail address:
....

Name:
....

Phone number:
....

Emergency phone number:
....

Address:
....

....

E-mail address:
....

Name:
....

Phone number:
....

Emergency phone number:
....

Address:
....

....

E-mail address:
....

Name:
....

Phone number:
....

Emergency phone number:
....

Address:
....

....

E-mail address:
....

Name:
....

Phone number:
....

Emergency phone number:
....

Address:
....

....

E-mail address:
....

Name:
....

Phone number:
....

Emergency phone number:
....

Address:
....

....

E-mail address:
....

Name:
....

Phone number:
....

Emergency phone number:
....

Address:
....

....

E-mail address:
....

Name:
....

Phone number:
....

Emergency phone number:
....

Address:
....

....

E-mail address:
....

Name:
....

Phone number:
....

Emergency phone number:
....

Address:
....

....

E-mail address:
....

Name:
....

Phone number:
....

Emergency phone number:
....

Address:
....

....

E-mail address:
....

Name:
....

Phone number:
....

Emergency phone number:
....

Address:
....

....

E-mail address:
....

Appendix B: Important Contact Information

Name:

Phone number:

Emergency phone number:

Address:

E-mail address:

Name:

Phone number:

Emergency phone number:

Address:

E-mail address:

Name:

Phone number:

Emergency phone number:

Address:

E-mail address:

Name:
....

Phone number:
....

Emergency phone number:
....

Address:
....

....

E-mail address:
....

Name:
....

Phone number:
....

Emergency phone number:
....

Address:
....

....

E-mail address:
....

Name:
....

Phone number:
....

Emergency phone number:
....

Address:
....

....

E-mail address:
....

Name:
....

Phone number:
....

Emergency phone number:
....

Address:
....

....

E-mail address:
....

Name:
....

Phone number:
....

Emergency phone number:
....

Address:
....

....

E-mail address:
....

Name:
....

Phone number:
....

Emergency phone number:
....

Address:
....

....

E-mail address:
....

Name:
....

Phone number:
....

Emergency phone number:
....

Address:
....

....

E-mail address:
....

Name:
....

Phone number:
....

Emergency phone number:
....

Address:
....

....

E-mail address:
....

Name:
....

Phone number:
....

Emergency phone number:
....

Address:
....

....

E-mail address:
....

Name:
....

Phone number:
....

Emergency phone number:
....

Address:
....

....

E-mail address:
....

Name:
....

Phone number:
....

Emergency phone number:
....

Address:
....

....

E-mail address:
....

Name:
....

Phone number:
....

Emergency phone number:
....

Address:
....

....

E-mail address:
....

Appendix B: Important Contact Information

Name:

Phone number:

Emergency phone number:

Address:

E-mail address:

Name:

Phone number:

Emergency phone number:

Address:

E-mail address:

Name:

Phone number:

Emergency phone number:

Address:

E-mail address:

APPENDIX C

Ten-Month Calendar

Use this calendar to track prenatal appointments, pregnancy milestones, and other important dates. You can also use it to record what you eat to ensure that you are getting a balanced diet and enough calories as your pregnancy progresses.

How to Set Up Your Calendar

Start the calendar with the first day of your last period, even if it didn't fall on the first day of the month. This is an important date to remember; your doctor will require it to determine your due date.

Next, count out forty weeks—or 280 days—from the first day of your last period. This will be your "due date." In most pregnancies it is almost impossible to determine the exact moment of conception, and this is the best way doctors can approximate when you will deliver. Mark this date on the calendar; it should fall on the very last page.

In between, fill out the months and days. While the calendar will look different than a standard calendar, to you it will serve a much more important function. And toward the end of your pregnancy, you'll surely be counting the days until the baby arrives.

Month .... *Week* ....

Monday

Tuesday

Wednesday

Thursday

Friday

Saturday

Sunday

Month

Week

Monday

Tuesday

Wednesday

Thursday

Friday

Saturday

Sunday

Monday

Tuesday

Wednesday

Thursday

Friday

Saturday

Sunday

Monday

Tuesday

Wednesday

Thursday

Friday

Saturday

Sunday

Monday

Tuesday

Wednesday

Thursday

Friday

Saturday

Sunday

Monday

Tuesday

Wednesday

Thursday

Friday

Saturday   Sunday

Monday

Tuesday

Wednesday

Thursday

Friday

Saturday

Sunday

Monday

Tuesday

Wednesday

Thursday

Friday

Saturday

Sunday

....
Month

....
Week

Monday

Tuesday

Wednesday

Thursday

Friday

Saturday

Sunday

Monday

Tuesday

Wednesday

Thursday

Friday

Saturday   Sunday

Monday

Tuesday

Wednesday

Thursday

Friday

Saturday

Sunday

Month

Week

Monday

Tuesday

Wednesday

Thursday

Friday

Saturday

Sunday

....

Month

....

Week

Monday

Tuesday

Wednesday

Thursday

Friday

Saturday

Sunday

Monday

Tuesday

Wednesday

Thursday

Friday

Saturday

Sunday

Month

....

Week

Monday

Tuesday

Wednesday

Thursday

Friday

Saturday

Sunday

Monday

Tuesday

Wednesday

Thursday

Friday

Saturday

Sunday

Monday

Tuesday

Wednesday

Thursday

Friday

Saturday   Sunday

Monday

Tuesday

Wednesday

Thursday

Friday

Saturday

Sunday

Monday

Tuesday

Wednesday

Thursday

Friday

Saturday

Sunday

Month ....

Week ....

Monday

Tuesday

Wednesday

Thursday

Friday

Saturday

Sunday

Monday

Tuesday

Wednesday

Thursday

Friday

Saturday

Sunday

Monday

Tuesday

Wednesday

Thursday

Friday

Saturday

Sunday

....

Month

....

Week

○ Monday

○ Tuesday

○ Wednesday

○ Thursday

○ Friday

○ Saturday

○ Sunday

Monday

Tuesday

Wednesday

Thursday

Friday

Saturday

Sunday

Month

Week

◯ Monday

◯ Tuesday

◯ Wednesday

◯ Thursday

◯ Friday

◯ Saturday

◯ Sunday

....
Month

....
Week

Monday

Tuesday

Wednesday

Thursday

Friday

Saturday

Sunday

274

Monday

Tuesday

Wednesday

Thursday

Friday

Saturday

Sunday

....

Month   *Week*

Monday

Tuesday

Wednesday

Thursday

Friday

Saturday   Sunday

Month

Week

Monday

Tuesday

Wednesday

Thursday

Friday

Saturday

Sunday

.... *Month*

.... *Week*

Monday

Tuesday

Wednesday

Thursday

Friday

Saturday

Sunday

Monday

Tuesday

Wednesday

Thursday

Friday

Saturday

Sunday

Monday

Tuesday

Wednesday

Thursday

Friday

Saturday

Sunday

....
Month

....
Week

Monday

Tuesday

Wednesday

Thursday

Friday

Saturday

Sunday

Monday

Tuesday

Wednesday

Thursday

Friday

Saturday

Sunday

Monday

Tuesday

Wednesday

Thursday

Friday

Saturday

Sunday

Monday

Tuesday

Wednesday

Thursday

Friday

Saturday

Sunday

Month

Week

Monday

Tuesday

Wednesday

Thursday

Friday

Saturday

Sunday

Month

Week

Monday

Tuesday

Wednesday

Thursday

Friday

Saturday

Sunday

Month

....

Week

Monday

Tuesday

Wednesday

Thursday

Friday

Saturday

Sunday

APPENDIX D

Estimated Due Date Table

ESTIMATED DUE DATE TABLE

DATE OF LAST PERIOD	YOUR EDD	DATE OF LAST PERIOD	YOUR EDD
1/1	10/8	2/7	11/14
1/2	10/9	2/8	11/15
1/3	10/10	2/9	11/16
1/4	10/11	2/10	11/17
1/5	10/12	2/11	11/18
1/6	10/13	2/12	11/19
1/7	10/14	2/13	11/20
1/8	10/15	2/14	11/21
1/9	10/16	2/15	11/22
1/10	10/17	2/16	11/23
1/11	10/18	2/17	11/24
1/12	10/19	2/18	11/25
1/13	10/20	2/19	11/26
1/14	10/21	2/20	11/27
1/15	10/22	2/21	11/28
1/16	10/23	2/22	11/29
1/17	10/24	2/23	11/30
1/18	10/25	2/24	12/1
1/19	10/26	2/25	12/2
1/20	10/27	2/26	12/3
1/21	10/28	2/27	12/4
1/22	10/29	2/28	12/5
1/23	10/30	**3/1**	12/6
1/24	10/31	3/2	12/7
1/25	11/1	3/3	12/8
1/26	11/2	3/4	12/9
1/27	11/3	3/5	12/10
1/28	11/4	3/6	12/11
1/29	11/5	3/7	12/12
1/30	11/6	3/8	12/13
1/31	11/7	3/9	12/14
2/1	11/8	3/10	12/15
2/2	11/9	3/11	12/16
2/3	11/10	3/12	12/17
2/4	11/11	3/13	12/18
2/5	11/12	3/14	12/19
2/6	11/13	3/15	12/20

ESTIMATED DUE DATE TABLE

DATE OF LAST PERIOD	YOUR EDD	DATE OF LAST PERIOD	YOUR EDD
3/16	12/21	4/22	1/27
3/17	12/22	4/23	1/28
3/18	12/23	4/24	1/29
3/19	12/24	4/25	1/30
3/20	12/25	4/26	1/31
3/21	12/26	4/27	2/1
3/22	12/27	4/28	2/2
3/23	12/28	4/29	2/3
3/24	12/29	4/30	2/4
3/25	12/30	**5/1**	2/5
3/26	12/31	5/2	2/6
3/27	1/1	5/3	2/7
3/28	1/2	5/4	2/8
3/29	1/3	5/5	2/9
3/30	1/4	5/6	2/10
3/31	1/5	5/7	2/11
4/1	1/6	5/8	2/12
4/2	1/7	5/9	2/13
4/3	1/8	5/10	2/14
4/4	1/9	5/11	2/15
4/5	1/10	5/12	2/16
4/6	1/11	5/13	2/17
4/7	1/12	5/14	2/18
4/8	1/13	5/15	2/19
4/9	1/14	5/16	2/20
4/10	1/15	5/17	2/21
4/11	1/16	5/18	2/22
4/12	1/17	5/19	2/23
4/13	1/18	5/20	2/24
4/14	1/19	5/21	2/25
4/15	1/20	5/22	2/26
4/16	1/21	5/23	2/27
4/17	1/22	5/24	2/28
4/18	1/23	5/25	3/1
4/19	1/24	5/26	3/2
4/20	1/25	5/27	3/3
4/21	1/26	5/28	3/4

ESTIMATED DUE DATE TABLE

DATE OF LAST PERIOD	YOUR EDD	DATE OF LAST PERIOD	YOUR EDD
5/29	3/5	7/5	4/11
5/30	3/6	7/6	4/12
5/31	3/7	7/7	4/13
6/1	3/8	7/8	4/14
6/2	3/9	7/9	4/15
6/3	3/10	7/10	4/16
6/4	3/11	7/11	4/17
6/5	3/12	7/12	4/18
6/6	3/13	7/13	4/19
6/7	3/14	7/14	4/20
6/8	3/15	7/15	4/21
6/9	3/16	7/16	4/22
6/10	3/17	7/17	4/23
6/11	3/18	7/18	4/24
6/12	3/19	7/19	4/25
6/13	3/20	7/20	4/26
6/14	3/21	7/21	4/27
6/15	3/22	7/22	4/28
6/16	3/23	7/23	4/29
6/17	3/24	7/24	4/30
6/18	3/25	7/25	5/1
6/19	3/26	7/26	5/2
6/20	3/27	7/27	5/3
6/21	3/28	7/28	5/4
6/22	3/29	7/29	5/5
6/23	3/30	7/30	5/6
6/24	3/31	7/31	5/7
6/25	4/1	**8/1**	5/8
6/26	4/2	8/2	5/9
6/27	4/3	8/3	5/10
6/28	4/4	8/4	5/11
6/29	4/5	8/5	5/12
6/30	4/6	8/6	5/13
7/1	4/7	8/7	5/14
7/2	4/8	8/8	5/15
7/3	4/9	8/9	5/16
7/4	4/10	8/10	5/17

ESTIMATED DUE DATE TABLE

DATE OF LAST PERIOD	YOUR EDD	DATE OF LAST PERIOD	YOUR EDD
8/11	5/18	9/17	6/24
8/12	5/19	9/18	6/25
8/13	5/20	9/19	6/26
8/14	5/21	9/20	6/27
8/15	5/22	9/21	6/28
8/16	5/23	9/22	6/29
8/17	5/24	9/23	6/30
8/18	5/25	9/24	7/1
8/19	5/26	9/25	7/2
8/20	5/27	9/26	7/3
8/21	5/28	9/27	7/4
8/22	5/29	9/28	7/5
8/23	5/30	9/29	7/6
8/24	5/31	9/30	7/7
8/25	6/1	**10/1**	7/8
8/26	6/2	10/2	7/9
8/27	6/3	10/3	7/10
8/28	6/4	10/4	7/11
8/29	6/5	10/5	7/12
8/30	6/6	10/6	7/13
8/31	6/7	10/7	7/14
9/1	6/8	10/8	7/15
9/2	6/9	10/9	7/16
9/3	6/10	10/10	7/17
9/4	6/11	10/11	7/18
9/5	6/12	10/12	7/19
9/6	6/13	10/13	7/20
9/7	6/14	10/14	7/21
9/8	6/15	10/15	7/22
9/9	6/16	10/16	7/23
9/10	6/17	10/17	7/24
9/11	6/18	10/18	7/25
9/12	6/19	10/19	7/26
9/13	6/20	10/20	7/27
9/14	6/21	10/21	7/28
9/15	6/22	10/22	7/29
9/16	6/23	10/23	7/30

ESTIMATED DUE DATE TABLE

DATE OF LAST PERIOD	YOUR EDD	DATE OF LAST PERIOD	YOUR EDD
10/24	7/31	11/28	9/4
10/25	8/1	11/29	9/5
10/26	8/2	11/30	9/6
10/27	8/3	**12/1**	9/7
10/28	8/4	12/2	9/8
10/29	8/5	12/3	9/9
10/30	8/6	12/4	9/10
10/31	8/7	12/5	9/11
11/1	8/8	12/6	9/12
11/2	8/9	12/7	9/13
11/3	8/10	12/8	9/14
11/4	8/11	12/9	9/15
11/5	8/12	12/10	9/16
11/6	8/13	12/11	9/17
11/7	8/14	12/12	9/18
11/8	8/15	12/13	9/19
11/9	8/16	12/14	9/20
11/10	8/17	12/15	9/21
11/11	8/18	12/16	9/22
11/12	8/19	12/17	9/23
11/13	8/20	12/18	9/24
11/14	8/21	12/19	9/25
11/15	8/22	12/20	9/26
11/16	8/23	12/21	9/27
11/17	8/24	12/22	9/28
11/18	8/25	12/23	9/29
11/19	8/26	12/24	9/30
11/20	8/27	12/25	10/1
11/21	8/28	12/26	10/2
11/22	8/29	12/27	10/3
11/23	8/30	12/28	10/4
11/24	8/31	12/29	10/5
11/25	9/1	12/30	10/6
11/26	9/2	12/31	10/7
11/27	9/3		